CW00924894

Contents

Foreword

Professor T. Colin Campbell

There is hardly another controversy in health science more contentious than the role of cow's milk and its products in our daily diet. Some wonder why we would even dare to question whether there are adverse health effects. For them, cow's milk is Nature's most perfect food. It builds strong bones and teeth and is a good source of calcium and protein.

Besides, it represents a bucolic side of life where gentle, lowing cows, black and white, roam in lush green pastures. I know this, for I was raised on a family dairy farm, milking cows and walking those green pastures, then combining grain and putting up hay for the winter. I drank the milk, lots of it, and we often made our own ice-cream and butter.

Early in my research career at Massachusetts Institute of Technology and Virginia Tech, I worked to promote better health by eating more meat, milk and eggs, what I believed to be 'high-quality animal protein'. It was an obvious sequel to my own life on the farm and I was happy to believe that the American diet was the best in the world.

However, later I was the Campus Coordinator at Virginia Tech of a project in the Philippines working with malnourished children. The primary goal of the project was to ensure that the children were getting as much protein as possible.

In this project, however, I observed something quite unusual. Children who ate the highest protein diets – and particularly animal protein – were the ones most likely to get liver cancer. I began to review other reports from around the world that reflected the findings of my research in the Philippines.

Although it was heretical to say that animal protein wasn't healthy, I started an in-depth study into the role of nutrition in the cause of cancer.
The research project culminated in a 20-year partnership of Cornell University, Oxford University, and the Chinese Academy of Preventive Medicine, a survey of diseases and lifestyle factors in rural China and Taiwan. More commonly known as the *China Study*, this project eventually produced more than 8,000 statistically significant associations between various dietary factors and disease.

This opportunity arose from a Chinese government

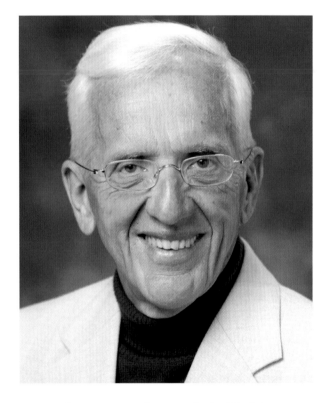

survey of cancer mortality rates in 2,400 Chinese counties that showed remarkable concentrations of cancer in certain counties and much less so in others. We then organised an additional and unusually comprehensive and unique survey of diet and lifestyle characteristics that might help to explain these unusual geographic concentrations of cancer. Personally, I was interested in the broad based hypothesis that animal and plant-based foods, as characterised by their nutrient profiles, have opposing effects on the chronic, so-called Western diseases like cancer.

The results from this massive study, when considered in relation to our earlier research and that of others, convinced me that the diet having the broadest range of health benefits is one that is comprised of a variety of whole plant-based foods, but one that is also low in added fat, salt, sugar and highly processed foods. Remarkably, relatively low intakes of animal-based foods (such as dairy products and meat) in rural China were associated with biological conditions that favour the occurrence of the chronic diseases typically found in Western industrialised countries.

Then it was on to discovering how broad might be this dietary effect. My son, Tom, and I turned our attention to the research investigations of others.

The published literature of these investigations is unimaginably huge. Moreover, the breadth of the health benefits of a plant-based diet is even far greater than our own research had indicated, with it reducing the risk of additional cancers, various cardiovascular diseases, diabetes (types I and II), multiple autoimmune diseases, osteoporosis, psycho-neural diseases (eg attention deficit disorder, clinical depression, Alzheimer's, cognitive dysfunction), eye disorders, kidney diseases, skin ailments and obesity amongst others.

Importantly, animal-based foods, as a group, have substantially different nutritional characteristics from plant-based foods and it is these nutritional characteristics, highly integrated at the metabolic level, that are chiefly responsible for the opposing effects of plant and animal-based foods on health and disease. Moreover, these effects involve countless food chemicals and exist throughout the range of consumption of these foods.

Of course, dairy foods have nutritional characteristics and disease associations that are consistent with other animal-based foods. Indeed, if anything, cow's milk and its products appear to be even more problematic than other animal-based foods.

Unfortunately the scientific literature on the characteristics and associations of dairy with health and disease seem to have been more obscured from public view than is the case for other animal-based foods. For example, research 40-60 years ago had shown that cow's milk proteins (casein and lactalbumin) markedly elevated blood cholesterol and its parallel formation of atherosclerotic plaques. More recently, much more evidence on the adverse health effects of cow's milk have accumulated, and much of it has been ably reviewed in this excellent report which is timely, broad in scope and profound in its consistency.

And finally, two other observations need attention. First, it is likely that the adverse dairy effects observed in many studies are underestimated because they have been observed in humans where the dairy-like nutritional effect already has been maximised by other animal-based foods. Second, imprecise measurement of risk factors and outcomes will mathematically attenuate the real effect.

It is not that these various dairy effects are independently proven to be true beyond doubt, any more than tobacco use is independently proven to cause lung cancer and heart disease. Rather, it is the weight and breadth of the evidence, along with its biological plausibility, that should determine the reliability of the evidence. Using these criteria, there is no doubt that this evidence on dairy is sufficient, at a minimum, to question the rather specious claims of health for cow's milk that have been made by the industry and its supporters and apologists.

I know well that this information deeply troubles many people, as it did me. But, at some point, we must give public voice to these observations and, if necessary, to sponsor discourse that is candid, openly transparent and, as much as possible, free of commercial bias.

T. Colin Campbell, PhD
Jacob Gould Schurman Professor Emeritus of Nutritional Biochemistry
Cornell University, Ithaca, NY
February 2014

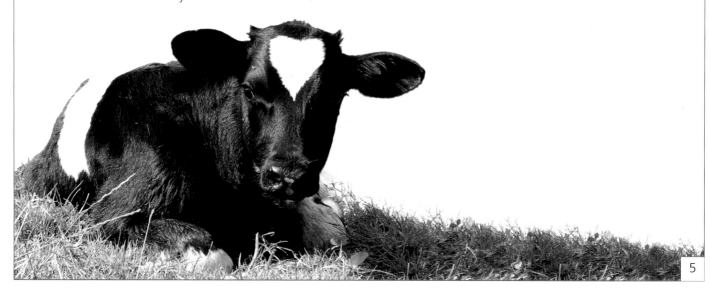

Foreword

Professor Jane Plant CBE (DSc)

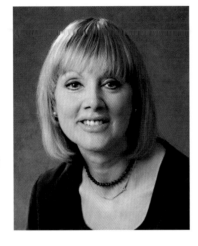

I was delighted to be asked to write a foreword for this excellent and well-researched report into the adverse health impacts of dairy consumption on human health. My book, *Your Life in Your Hands*, describes how giving up dairy produce has helped me and other women to overcome metastatic breast cancer. When it was first published in 2000, I faced a barrage of criticism from orthodox doctors, charities and nutritionists. All of them, for whatever reason, poured scorn on the idea that consuming dairy could be bad for health. This may have been because, as Dr Justine Butler shows in this report, we have all been subjected to relentless publicity from the industry that tries to persuade us that dairy is wholesome, natural and good for our health. It is a measure of how far medical opinion has changed that in 2005 I was awarded a life fellowship of the Royal Society of Medicine in recognition of my contribution to science through my books. We have a long way to go, however, until the truth about dairy is generally accepted, so this report is both timely and very welcome.

When I was carrying out the research for *Your Life in Your Hands*, which includes more than 500 references from the peer reviewed scientific literature, I was astonished at just how much information was available on the role of dairy produce in promoting disease – not only breast, prostate, ovarian and other cancers but also other conditions ranging from eczema and other allergic conditions to heart disease and diabetes. Despite all the criticism of my books, no one has presented a single scientific fact that persuades me to change one sentence of what I wrote in 2000 – and as a trained scientist I would have done that had I been given convincing evidence that I was wrong or had misunderstood some issue. Instead, the evidence against consuming dairy produce has continued to mount, as I detailed in the second and third editions of *Your Life in Your Hands*, and in my other books,

Prostate Cancer, Osteoporosis (yes – there is even a compelling case against dairy produce, especially cheese, in the development of this crippling bone disease) and *Eating for Better Health*. This new report takes the evidence on the adverse human health impacts of dairy further.

What I had not appreciated until I attended the excellent and thought-provoking lecture given by Juliet Gellatley of Viva! at the Incredible Veggie Show in London in 2005 was the true nature of the modern dairy industry. It is hard to forget some of the images of cruelty that she presented then. This report exposes the nature of the modern industrialised dairy industry and the serious implications that this has for our health. I do hope that *White Lies* receives the recognition it deserves and that this will embolden politicians to take a stand against the dairy industry. To do so would improve human health, improve the environment, address serious issues of animal welfare and save the taxpayer a great deal of money spent in subsidising an industry that was the centre of the BSE crisis, the foot and mouth disease disaster and now the bovine tuberculosis problem.

Cow's milk is a perfect food for a rapidly growing calf but that doesn't mean it is good for human babies – or adults! If you want to improve your health by making just one change to your diet, I recommend you eliminate all dairy from the diet.

Professor Jane Plant CBE (DSc, CEng)
Life Fellow of the Royal Society of Medicine
Professor of Applied Geochemistry
Imperial College, London
February 2014

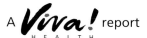
Introduction

The foods we consume are of immense importance to our health and well-being. The recent increase in television and media coverage of food and health issues has improved our understanding of the links that exist between diet and health. The types of food that we eat are strongly linked to our culture and food issues can cause emotional responses. In the UK and other northern European countries as well as North America, we have developed a strong emotional attachment to the idea that milk is a natural and healthy drink for us, even as adults.

Milk is the first food that we consume, our mother's breast milk if we are fortunate, if not then specially formulated substitutes based on cow's or soya milk are generally used in the UK. We associate milk with comfort and nurturing and consider milk to be a wholesome nutrient-rich component of the diet that is essential for normal growth and development, which for a baby it is. However, all other mammals on the planet are weaned off milk at an early age, whereas some humans continue drinking milk into adulthood. Not only that, we drink the milk of another species, something no other mammal does. To be fair, contrary to popular belief, most people in the world do not drink milk; it would make many of us ill. But in the UK, we are a nation of milk drinkers, along with most other northern European countries and North America. Infants, the young, adolescents, adults and the aged all consume large quantities of milk, cheese, butter and yogurt every year. But why are we so convinced that milk is some kind of wonder food?

Milk, it seems, can help you lose weight; it can also make you gain weight. Milk promotes healthy skin; it may also cause acne. You need milk for good bone health, but the incidence of osteoporosis is highest in countries that consume the most milk. These conflicting reports leave us confused and unsure who to believe. The dairy industry invests millions in milk advertising and promotion. It could be argued that they present a biased view motivated by financial interest. An increasing amount of scientific evidence now shows that cow's milk is not the wonder food the dairy industry would have us believe. This research goes further in linking the consumption of cow's milk to a wide range of health problems. Many people, even health professionals, may find it hard to be objective about the detrimental impact of dairy products on health described in this report because of the emotional attachment many of us have to the idea that milk is natural and healthy.

The aim of this report is to redress the balance by presenting and reviewing the research on the health effects of cow's milk and dairy products.

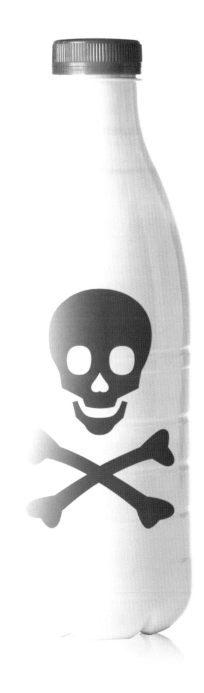

What is a healthy diet?

A healthy diet contains a wide range of fresh fruit and vegetables, whole grains, pulses, nuts and seeds. It is rich in important fibre and disease-busting antioxidants that protect against a number of illnesses and diseases including certain cancers and cardiovascular disease (Genkinger *et al.*, 2004; He *et al.*, 2007; Rautiainen *et al.*, 2012). It has been suggested that the high concentration of antioxidants in blood may be one of the reasons for the lower incidence of chronic diseases in people consuming a plant-based diet rich in fruit and vegetables (Waldman *et al.*, 2005). A healthy diet provides plenty of fibre protecting against a range of diseases including colorectal cancer (Murphy *et al.* 2012). It is rich in vitamins and minerals, again protecting health. A healthy diet should contain a good source of plant-based essential polyunsaturated fatty acids including the omega-3 fatty acids known to protect heart health (Pan *et al.*, 2012).

On the other hand, a healthy diet should be low in saturated fat, animal protein and cholesterol for which we have no dietary requirement. Too much saturated fat can increase the amount of cholesterol in the blood, which increases your risk of developing heart disease. Saturated fat is found in many foods, such as hard cheese, cakes, biscuits, sausages, cream, butter, lard and pies. The government recommends that we eat less of these types of food and choose foods that contain unsaturated rather than saturated fats (NHS Choices, 2012). This means eating more avocados, nuts and seeds and plant-based oils and spreads such as flax seed oil and soya spread.

Cow's milk, cheese, butter, cream, ice-cream and milk chocolate all contain the unhealthy saturated kind of fat associated with an increased risk of heart disease. Some of these foods contain considerable amounts of saturated fat. For example, Cheddar cheese contains around 35 per cent fat, of which over 60 per cent is saturated. Similarly, butter contains over 80 per cent fat, of which over 60 per cent is saturated (FSA, 2002). This means that a 10 gram serving of butter contains over five grams of saturated fat! The Government provide guidelines to tell you if a food is high or low in total and saturated fat (see Table 1).

So the five grams of saturated fat contained in just 10 grams of butter makes this food remarkably unhealthy. Plant-based polyunsaturated fat spreads contain less total fat (around 60 per cent) of which less than 20 per cent is saturated. They tend to contain more of the valuable polyunsaturated fatty acids and so provide a much healthier option.

Table 1 Government guidelines on fat content

Total fat

More than 17.5g of fat per 100g	High
3g of fat or less per 100g	Low

Saturated fat

More than 5g of saturated fat per 100g	High
1.5g of saturated fat or less per 100g	Low

Source: NHS Choices, 2013.

Saturated fats from animal foods such as whole milk, cream and butter increase the amount of cholesterol in the blood which in turn increases the risk of heart disease and diabetes. Research shows that a plant-based diet contains significantly less saturated fat. The extensive EPIC Oxford study comprising 33,883 meat-eaters, 10,110 fish-eaters, 18,840 vegetarians and 2,596 vegans showed that while the total fat intake was highest in the meat-eaters and lowest in vegans, the difference between the groups was relatively small. However, the percentage of energy from saturated fat was strikingly different across the four diet groups: saturated fat intake was highest in meat-eaters, almost identical in fish-eaters and vegetarians and significantly lowest among the vegans (Davey *et al.*, 2003). So significant is the lower saturated fat content of a plant-based diet that it can be used to control weight without worrying about calorie counting. In one clinical trial, adoption of a low-fat vegan diet was shown to help weight loss despite the absence of prescribed limits on portion size or energy intake (Barnard *et al.*, 2005). Other research confirming that vegetarians and vegans have a lower risk of overweight and obesity than meat-eaters shows that consuming more plant foods and less animal products may help individuals control their weight (Newby, *et al.*, 2005). Being overweight or obese increases the risk of many health problems including type 2 diabetes, heart disease, asthma, infertility, high blood pressure and many cancers.

Milk and other dairy products contain many biologically active molecules including hormones and growth factors. Cow's milk has been shown to contain over 35 different hormones and 11 growth factors (Grosvenor *et al.*, 1992). Some researchers are particularly concerned about the oestrogen content of cow's milk (Ganmaa and Sato, 2005),

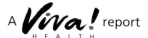

suggesting that cow's milk is one of the important routes of human exposure to oestrogens. The milk consumed now is very different to the milk consumed a century ago. Unlike their pasture-fed counterparts of old, modern dairy cows are usually pregnant and continue to lactate during the latter half of pregnancy, when the concentration of oestrogens in blood, and hence in the milk, increases. Although there is a paucity of research in this field, early evidence suggests the increase in exposure to cow's oestrogen may be linked to an increased incidence of certain cancers. In one study, cancer incidence was correlated with food intake in 40 countries (Ganmaa and Sato, 2005). Results showed that both cow's milk and cheese increased the risk of hormone-dependent cancers such as breast and ovarian cancer. Among the dietary risk factors identified, these researchers were most concerned with milk and dairy products because, as already stated, the milk drunk today tends to come from pregnant cows among whom oestrogen and progesterone levels are markedly elevated.

Another bioactive component of cow's milk receiving an increasing amount of attention is the growth factor called insulin-like growth factor 1 (IGF-1). The amount of IGF-1 present is higher in milk produced by pregnant cows. The concern is that because IGF-1 in cows is identical to human IGF-1, this growth factor could cross the gut wall and trigger an abnormal response, for example increasing the risk of certain cancers. It may be that IGF-1 does not cross the gut wall but that other bioactive components in milk boost IGF-1 production in the liver (see IGF-1). Either way, over the last decade IGF-1 has been linked to an increased risk of childhood cancers, breast cancer, lung cancer, melanoma and cancers of the pancreas and prostate (LeRoith *et al.*, 1995; Chan *et al.*, 1998) and gastrointestinal cancers (Epstein, 1996).

Interestingly, one study observed a 10 per cent increase in blood serum levels of IGF-1 in subjects who increased their intake of non-fat milk (Heaney, 1999) while another study noted that vegan men had a nine per cent lower serum IGF-1 level than meat-eaters and vegetarians (Allen *et al.*, 2000). Whether the consumption of cow's milk and dairy products raises IGF-1 levels directly (by crossing the gut wall), or indirectly (by triggering an increased production of human IGF-1 in the body), evidence suggests that some component of milk causes an increase in blood serum levels of IGF-1. It has even been suggested that IGF-1 may be used as a predictor of certain cancers, in much the same way that cholesterol is a predictor of heart disease (Campbell and Campbell, 2005).

In summary, a diet containing saturated fat, cholesterol, animal protein, hormones and growth factors is not a healthy diet. Cow's milk, butter, cheese, cream, ice-cream and other dairy products contain all these unhealthy components whereas substantial evidence shows that a plant-based diet rich in fruit and vegetables, whole grains and unsaturated fats (including omega-3 fatty acids) offers significant health benefits. By adopting a healthy diet, together with regular physical exercise, avoiding smoking and drinking (alcohol) only moderately, many of the so-called modern Western diseases can be prevented. As part of its global strategy on diet, physical activity and health, the World Health Organisation (WHO) claims that up to 80 per cent of cases of coronary heart disease, 90 per cent of type 2 diabetes cases and one-third of cancers can be avoided by changing to a healthier diet, increasing physical activity and stopping smoking (WHO, 2003).

Part one:
The History, Geography and Biology of Milk

The Origins of Dairy Farming

Although sheep, cattle and goats are thought to have been domesticated in parts of the Middle East and central Asia over 9,000 years ago there is no direct evidence that these animals were used to supply milk. Written texts, paintings and drawings from around 6,000 years ago provide evidence of dairy farming from then (Pringle, 1998). However, analysis of dairy fat residues on pottery fragments suggests that the exploitation of animals for milk was already an established practice in Britain when farming began in the fifth millennium BC (Copley *et al.*, 2003). More recent research show that humans in north-west Anatolia (Asia Minor or Turkey) were using milk 8,000 years ago (Evershed *et al.*, 2008). Analysis of fat residues on sieve-like pottery structures indicates that cheese manufacture may have been practiced by Neolithic people 7,500 years ago (Salque *et al.*, 2013).

The ability to digest lactose (the sugar in milk) evolved as a result of a genetic mutation among people in the Balkans and central Europe (amongst some other places) around 7,500 years ago. Descendants of these people are able to consume dairy milk today without suffering the symptoms of lactose intolerance (bloating, wind, discomfort etc). Cheese-making would have allowed the lactose-intolerant Neolithic farming communities to consume milk without becoming ill, as processing milk into cheese reduces the lactose content.

Although this all sounds like a long time ago, in evolutionary terms it is very recent history and early dairy farming would have been practised on a relatively small scale. Hominid (modern humans and our forerunners) fossils date back to nearly seven million years ago (Cela-Conde and Ayala, 2003). If seven million years were represented as a twelve-hour clock, starting at midday, humans would have started dairy farming less than one minute before midnight.

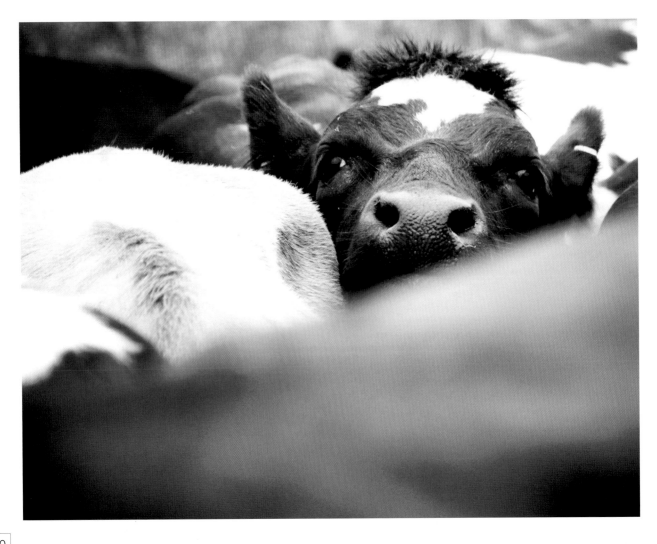

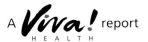

Dairy farming today

Milk production today is big business. The total value of the production of milk in the UK is estimated to be £3.8 billion (Defra, 2012). This is more than the value of production of beef, lamb, pig, poultry meat, eggs and around three times the value of the production of fresh vegetables (Defra, 2012).

There are now 1.81 million dairy cows in the UK dairy herd (Dairy Co, 2013). Although the numbers of dairy cows are falling year by year (down 7.3 per cent or 142,000 dairy cows in the last five years), the milk yield has increased. Defra states that the increase in milk yield far offsets the fall in the number of dairy cattle (Dairy Co, 2013a). The latest figures from Defra show that the total level of milk produced in the UK from 2011 to 2012 increased by 163 million litres to 13.8 billion litres (Dairy Co, 2013a). There is a clear trend; fewer cows are being forced to produce more milk.

Excluding suckled milk, each cow now produces over 20 litres of milk per day, which equates to 7,617 litres of milk yearly (Dairy Co, 2013a). Over the last 10 years, selective breeding and high protein feed has increased the average yield per cow from 17.7 litres per day to 20.9 litres per day. That is 3.2 litres additional milk being produced by dairy cows, every day!

A common misconception is that it is natural for cows to produce milk constantly. This is not the case; just like us, cows only produce milk after a nine-month pregnancy and giving birth. Today's large-scale intensive dairy farming employs a highly regulated regime of cycling pregnancy and lactation concurrently, meaning that cows are both pregnant and being milked at the same time for most of each year. This intensive physical demand puts a tremendous strain on the dairy cow and, as she gets older, infertility and severe infections causing mastitis and lameness cuts short her economic and productive life. The average lifespan of a modern dairy cow is only about five years – that is after three or four lactations, when naturally she may live for 20 to 30 years.

Who drinks milk?

Since 1960, global milk production has nearly doubled (Speedy, 2003). The most substantial growth has occurred in developing countries; the consumption of milk per person in China has increased tenfold since 1980 (FAO, 2009). These changes in diet have had an impact on the global demand for agricultural products and will continue to do so.

Around three-quarters of the world's population do not drink milk, but among those who do, the pattern of consumption varies widely between countries. Data collected by the Food and Agriculture Organisation of the United Nations (FAO) provides figures for the consumption of milk (excluding butter) in kilograms per capita per year for over 170 countries (FAOSTAT, 2013).

As shown in Figure 1.0 the level of milk and dairy product consumption varies widely between countries. The highest levels of consumption are seen in Europe. In Finland for example, a massive 375.4kg was consumed per person in 2009, with Sweden close behind at 357.4kg, then the Netherlands (357.3.7kg), Albania (282kg), Germany (264kg) and Norway (262.6kg). Between 2002 and 2009, US

Figure 1.0 Consumption of milk (excluding butter) in selected countries compared to world consumption.

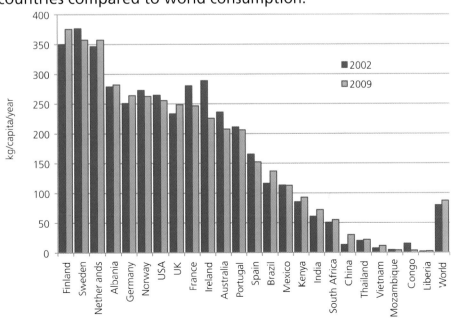

Data from FAOSTAT, 2013.

consumption dropped from 264.6kg to 255.6kg and UK consumption increased from 233.3kg to 248.5kg so the gap between the two has largely been closed. The average amount of milk and dairy products consumed per person per year on a global scale is just 87.3kg (up from 79.8kg in 2002). It should be noted that while overall dairy consumption in the UK may have increased, the consumption of milk in 2009 was reduced according to the 2008/2009 National Diet and Nutrition Survey. For example, consumption for girls aged 11-18 years was 136 grams per day on average in 1997 and 107grams per day in 2009; consumption for boys of the same age was 208 grams per day in 1997 and 172 grams per day in 2009. For adults, even larger decreases were seen, for women from 195 grams per day in 2000/2001 to 120 grams per day in 2009 and for men, from 225 grams per day to 165 grams per day (Bates *et al.*, 2010).

The lowest levels of consumption are seen in Africa and Asia. In Liberia a mere 2.5kg was consumed per person in 2009. Other countries consuming small amounts include the Congo (3.7kg), Mozambique (4.1kg), the Democratic People's Republic of Korea (4.5kg), Viet Nam (11.5kg) and Thailand (21.8kg). With levels this low, it is reasonable to assume that many people in these countries and others do not consume any milk or milk products at all.

While some European countries are consuming less (Sweden, France, Norway, Ireland, Portugal and Spain), consumption in developing countries is increasing (Brazil, Kenya, South Africa, India and China). In 2002 the amount consumed per person in China was 13.2kg, by 2009 this figured has risen to 29.8kg. Although the amount consumed per person in China is still relatively low compared to that in the West, it should be remembered that China has a population of 1.35 billion so this increase amounts to a significantly higher demand.

It could be argued that the lower level of consumption seen in some developing countries just reflects the fact that people cannot afford to buy milk products. However, in Japan for example (not a developing country), consumption is very low at only 73.9kg. Most people in the world do not drink milk; their reasons may be cultural, economic, historical or biological. For example, most of the world's population are lactose intolerant (see Lactose intolerance). But many of us think of milk as a fundamental component of a healthy diet. Why is this? Is milk the only source of some obscure essential nutrient? Or is milk unique in that it contains all the nutrients that we require?

A comparison between human milk and cow's milk

The composition of milk varies according to the animal from which it comes, providing the correct rate of growth and development for the young of that species, thus for human infants, human milk is obviously more suitable than cow's milk. Indeed, the popular consensus among health care professionals is that ordinary cow's milk, goat's milk, condensed milk, dried milk, evaporated milk, or any other type of milk should not be given to a child under the age of one. This is because of differences in the composition of milk that have been revealed by research over the last decade or so. While cow's milk and human milk contain a similar percentage of water, the relative amounts of carbohydrate, protein, fat, vitamins and minerals vary widely.

Figure 2.0 A comparison of the carbohydrate, protein and fat components of whole cow's milk and human milk.

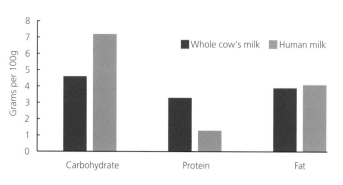

Source: FSA, 2002.

Protein
The carbohydrate, protein and fat content of milk from one species is finely tuned to meet the nutritional requirements of that particular animal whether human, elephant, buffalo, camel or dog. Figure 2.0 shows that the protein content in 100g of whole cow's milk (3.3g) is more than double that of human milk (1.3g); this is because the amount of protein in milk is linked to the amount of time it takes that particular species of animal to grow in size. Growing calves need more protein to enable them to grow quickly. Human infants on the other hand need less protein and more fat as their energies are expended primarily in the development of the brain, spinal cord and nerves.

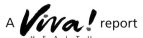
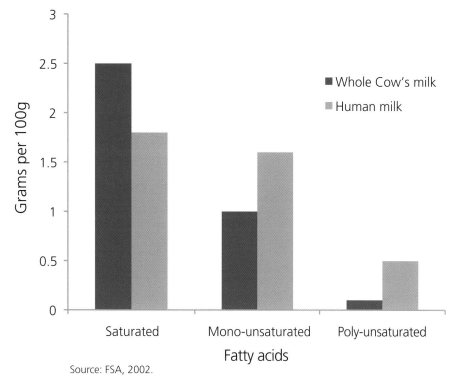

Figure 3.0 The fatty acid composition of whole cow's milk and human milk.

Source: FSA, 2002.

Species with the highest milk protein concentration exhibit the most rapid growth rate. Leucine is a unique amino acid in that it stimulates muscle protein synthesis. The higher the protein plus leucine content of milk, the quicker the neonate doubles its birth weight. For instance, the leucine content of rat's milk is 11 grams per litre and the rat doubles its birth weight in just four days. Cat's milk contains 8.9 grams per litre and the cat takes 10 days to double its birth weight. Cow's milk contains 3.3 grams per litre and the calf doubles its birth weight after 40 days. Human milk contains 0.9 grams per litre and the human infant, the mammal with the slowest growth rate, doubles its birth weight after 180 days. The weight gain of calves during the first year (0.7-0.8 kg per day) is nearly 40 times higher than that of breastfed human infants (0.02 kg per day). It has been demonstrated that cow's milk-based infant formula feeding significantly increases serum concentrations of leucine, insulin and IGF-1 in comparison to breast-feeding (Melnik *et al.*, 2012). This may be one of the mechanisms linking formula feeding to overweight and obesity (see Breast Is Best below).

The proteins in milk can be divided into two categories: caseins and whey proteins. Human milk contains these in a ratio of 40:60 respectively; while in cow's milk the ratio of casein to whey proteins is 80:20. Given that the amount of total protein in cow's milk is more than double that of human milk, cow's milk clearly contains considerably more casein than human milk. Casein can be difficult to digest, in fact it is used as the basis of some glues! Infant milks are formulated to contain more whey than casein (the ratio of whey to casein in these milks is similar to that of human milk), and this is why it is thought to be easier for new babies to digest. Casein has been linked to a range of diseases and allergies, including type 1 diabetes (see Diabetes).

Fat
The amount and type of fat present in the milk similarly reflects the requirements of the species of animal producing that milk. Whole milk from a cow

contains around four per cent fat whereas milk from the grey seal contains over 50 per cent fat (Baker, 1990); this is because baby seals need more body fat to survive in cold water. Figure 2.0 shows that 100g of whole cow's milk and human milk contain similar amounts of fat (3.9g and 4.1g respectively). While these values are close, the types of fat vary. Figure 3.0 shows that cow's milk contains more saturated fat while human milk contains more unsaturated fat.

Figure 3.0 shows that 100g of whole cow's milk contains 2.5g saturated fat, 1.0g monounsaturated and 0.1g polyunsaturated fat, while human milk contains 1.8g saturated fat, 1.6g monounsaturated fat and 0.5g polyunsaturated fat (FSA, 2002). These figures demonstrate the higher level of saturated fat in cow's milk compared to human milk, and the higher level of unsaturated fat in human milk compared to cow's milk. This imbalance contributes to the unsuitability of cow's milk for human infants.

The higher level of unsaturated fatty acids in human milk reflects the important role of these fats in brain development. In humans the brain develops rapidly during the first year of life, growing faster than the body and tripling in size by the age of one. The brain is largely composed of fat and early brain development and function in humans requires a sufficient supply of polyunsaturated essential fatty acids. The omega-6 fatty acid arachidonic acid (AA) and the omega-3 fatty acid docosahexaenoic acid (DHA) are both essential for brain development and functioning. Both are supplied in human milk but not in cow's milk (currently AA and DHA-enhanced infant formulas are available, although not mandatory, throughout most of Europe). Cow's milk does contain the shorter chain omega-6 linoleic acid (LNA) and the omega-3 α-linolenic acid (ALA) but these have to be converted in the body into the longer chain versions mentioned above.

A review of 20 studies of cognitive function of breast fed infants compared to that of formula fed infants concluded that the nutrients in breast milk may have a significant effect on neurological development in infants (Anderson *et al.*, 1999). More recent work indicates that compared to formula milk, nutrients in breast milk may confer better cognitive and motor development in infants (Bernard *et al.*, 2013) which may extend into intelligence in adulthood (Mortensen *et al.*, 2003).

Table 2.0 Comparison of the mineral and vitamin components of cow's milk and human milk.

	Cow's Milk (semi-skimmed, pasteurised) per 100g	Human Milk (mature) per 100g
Sodium (mg)	43	15
Potassium (mg)	156	58
Calcium (mg)	120	34
Magnesium (mg)	11	3
Phosphorus (mg)	94	15
Iron (mg)	0.02	0.07
Copper (mg)	Trace	0.04
Zinc (mg)	0.4	0.3
Chloride (mg)	87	42
Manganese (mg)	Trace	Trace
Selenium (g)	1	1
Iodine (g)	30	7
Retinol (g)	19	58
Carotene (g)	9	(24)
Vitamin D (g)	Trace	Trace
Vitamin E (mg)	0.04	0.34
Thiamin (mg)	0.03	0.02
Riboflavin (mg)	0.24	0.03
Niacin (mg)	0.1	0.2
Vitamin B6 (mg)	0.06	0.01
Vitamin B12 (g)	0.9	Trace
Folate (g)	9	5
Pantothenate (mg)	0.68	0.25
Biotin (g)	3.0	0.7
Vitamin C (mg)	2	4

( ) = estimated value. Source: FSA, 2002.

Cow's milk tends to be low in the types of fat essential for human brain development; a rapid increase in body size is more of an imperative for cows than rapid brain development, so cows produce milk that is high in body-building saturated fats to help their calves grow rapidly in size.

Similarly, the fatty acid composition of cow's milk is more suited to a calf than to a person. Attempts to alter the fatty acid composition of cow's milk, and so increase the nutritional value of cow's milk to humans, have involved experiments feeding cows fish meal and soya beans (AbuGhazaleh *et al.*, 2004) and flax seed (Petit, 2002). Feeding flax seed resulted in a lower omega-6 to omega-3 fatty acid ratio, which is thought might improve the nutritional value of milk from a human health point of view by reducing the potential risk of disease. Of course you could just eat the flax seed oil yourself to improve the balance of omega-3 and omega-6 oils in your diet while avoiding the undesirable components of milk.

Calcium
The calcium content of cow's milk (120mg per 100ml) is nearly four times that of human milk (34mg per 100ml). This discrepancy occurs for good reason;

calves grow much more quickly and have a larger skeleton than human babies and therefore need much more calcium (FAO, 1997). Cow's milk is specifically designed to meet this high demand which is why whole cow's milk is not recommended for infants under 12 months. Although human milk contains less calcium, it is more easily absorbed than that found in cow's milk. According to the American Academy of Pediatrics Committee on Nutrition, the available data demonstrate that the bioavailability of calcium from human milk is greater than that from infant formulas (58 per cent and 38 per cent respectively) (Greer and Krebs, 2006). In an effort to address this discrepancy, the concentration of calcium in infant formulas is generally higher than that in human milk. So although human milk contains less calcium than cow's milk, the calcium in human milk is better absorbed into the body than the calcium in cow's milk, again illustrating why human milk is the best source of nutrition during the first year of life.

Iron
Cow's milk contains very little iron (FSA, 2002) which is another reason why cow's milk is deemed to be unsuitable for infants under the age of 12 months. Indeed a one-year-old attempting to meet the

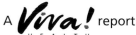
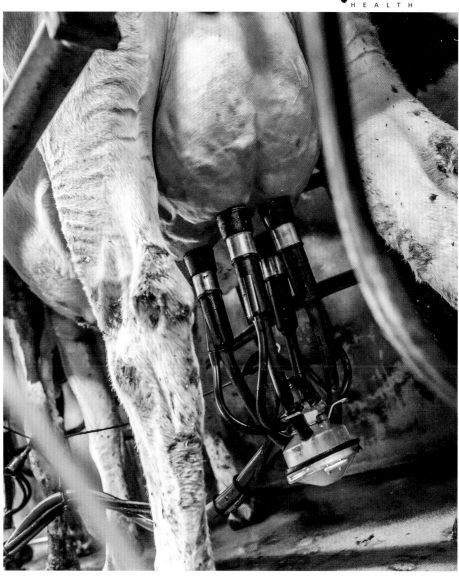

reference nutrient intake (RNI) of 5.3mg of iron would have to drink over 30 pints of cow's milk per day if it were to be used to meet their iron requirement. Furthermore, cow's milk is low in vitamin C and vitamin D (Department of Health, 1994), and contains less vitamin A than human milk.

The high protein, sodium, potassium, phosphorus and chloride content of cow's milk present what is called a high renal solute load; this means that the unabsorbed solutes from the diet must be excreted via the kidneys. This can place a strain on immature kidneys forcing them to draw water from the body thus increasing the risk of dehydration. The renal solute load of infants fed cow's milk has been shown to be twice as high as that of formula fed infants (Martinez *et al.*, 1985) and three times that of human milk (Ziegler, 2011).

Allergic reactions to the proteins in cow's milk are common among infants, and cow's milk-induced intestinal bleeding as an allergic response is a well-recognised cause of rectal bleeding in infancy (Willetts *et al.*, 1999). This blood loss can affect the iron nutritional status of the infant (Ziegler *et al.*, 2011) and in many cases may lead to anaemia. This condition will deteriorate if iron-rich foods are excluded by the continued consumption of milk, a food very low in iron (see Allergies – Gastrointestinal bleeding).

The health problems caused by the early consumption of 'normal' off-the-shelf cow's milk are so well documented that for some time now, parents and caregivers have been advised not to introduce cow's milk before the age of 12 months in the UK (Department of Health, 1994), the US (American Academy of Pediatrics, 1992), Denmark (The National Board of Health, Denmark, 1998) Canada (Canadian Paediatric Society, 1998), Sweden (Axelsson *et al.*, 1999) and New Zealand (Soh *et al.*, 2004).

The composition of cow's milk

Cow's milk composition can vary widely between different breeds and during different stages of lactation. In the first few days after birth, a special type of milk called colostrum is excreted which is rich in fats and protein. Colostrum also contains important infection-fighting antibodies which strengthen the immune system of the young mammal. The transition from colostrum to true milk occurs within a few days following birth.

Water
All milk produced by animals contains carbohydrate, protein, fat, minerals and vitamins but the major component is water. Water dilutes the milk allowing its secretion from the body; without water it would be impossible to express milk. Additionally, the water in milk is essential to the newborn for hydration. Cow's milk contains a similar amount of water to human milk – around 87 per cent.

Carbohydrate
The major carbohydrate in mammalian milk is a disaccharide (or sugar) called lactose. For lactose to

be digested, it must be broken down in the intestine by the enzyme lactase to its component monosaccharides glucose and galactose. Glucose can then supply energy to the young animal. Many people are unable to consume cow's milk and dairy products because they are unable to digest lactose after weaning. Most infants possess the enzyme lactase and can therefore digest lactose, but this ability is lost in many people after weaning (commonly after the age of two). In global terms lactose intolerance is very common, occurring in around 90-100 per cent of Asians, 65-70 per cent of Africans, but just 10 per cent of Caucasians (Robbins, 2001). **Therefore most of the world's population are unable to digest milk after weaning**.

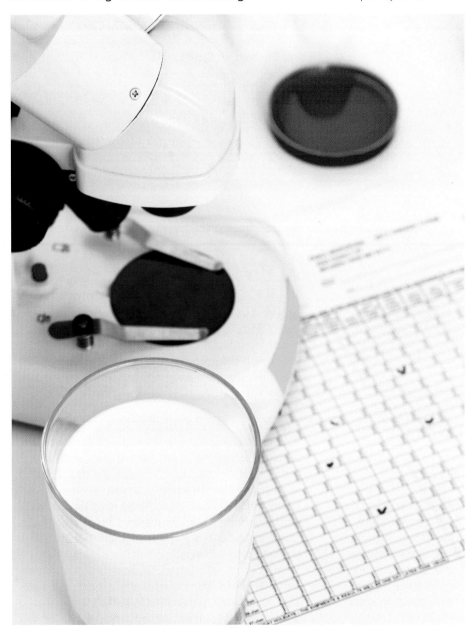

Protein

Protein provides energy and is required for the growth and repair of tissue such as skin and muscle. Caseins are the primary group of proteins in cow's milk, making up around 80 per cent of the total protein content. The remaining portion is made up from whey proteins. There are four types of casein (alpha$_{S1}$, alpha$_{S2}$, beta and kappa casein) that combine to make up a structure known as a casein micelle. The micellar structure of casein is important in the production of cheese; it also plays a significant role in cow's milk allergies (see Allergies).

Fat

The principal fat in milk is a complex combination of lipids called triglycerols (esters of three fatty acids with one molecule of glycerol). There are more than 400 fatty acids in cow's milk ranging in carbon atom chain length. Fatty acids are described as saturated or unsaturated depending on the amount of hydrogen in the carbon chain of the molecule; milk contains both saturated and unsaturated fatty acids. Unsaturated fatty acids may be further classified as monounsaturated or polyunsaturated (depending on the number of double bonds in the carbon chain of the fatty acid molecule). Most of the fat in whole cow's milk (around 65 per cent) is the saturated type. Around 30 per cent is monounsaturated and just five per cent polyunsaturated. Saturated fatty acids are associated with high blood cholesterol and heart disease.

Polyunsaturated fats include fatty acids called the omega-6 and omega-3 fatty acids, (these names refer to the position of the

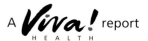
double bond in the carbon chain of the fatty acid molecule). Milk contains the omega-6 essential fatty acid linoleic acid and the omega-3 fatty acid linolenic acid. These are called essential fatty acids because they are essential to health but cannot be made within the body and so must be obtained from the diet. While milk does contain linoleic acid and linolenic acid (both with chains of 18 carbon atoms) it does so at relatively low levels.

There has been much excitement over the last ten years about conjugated linoleic acids (CLAs) in cow's milk. The term 'conjugated' refers to the molecular arrangement of the molecule. CLAs are described as positional and geometric isomers of linoleic acid; this means that CLAs are made up of exactly the same components as normal linoleic acid, just in a different arrangement. It has been suggested that some forms of CLA may confer a range of potential human health benefits (McGuire and McGuire, 2000, Whigham *et al.*, 2007). However, the majority of studies on weight loss, cancer, cardiovascular disease, insulin sensitivity and diabetes and immune function have been conducted on animals (or *in vitro*) and it has been acknowledged that variations exist between different animals' responses to CLAs. Human studies have produced mixed results; a review of 17 studies on humans concluded that CLA does not affect body weight or body composition and has a limited effect on immune function (Tricon *et al.*, 2005). Furthermore some detrimental effects of CLA have been observed in mice and some reports suggest that CLAs can elicit pro-carcinogenic effects (Wahle *et al.*, 2004). One form of CLA is suspected of having pro-diabetic effects in individuals who are already at risk of developing diabetes (McCrorie *et al.*, 2011).

In summary, there is no substantive evidence of a consistent benefit of CLA on any human health conditions and evidence regarding effectiveness of CLA in humans is inconclusive (Silveira *et al.*, 2007). Despite warnings from researchers that until we know more, CLA supplementation in humans should be considered with caution, the dairy industry sees this molecule as a new marketing opportunity and research into producing CLA-enriched milk, by manipulating the diet of dairy cows, began over a decade ago (Lock and Garnsworthy, 2002). As stated above, cow's milk and dairy products are significant source of saturated fat in the human diet. Altering the fatty acid composition of dairy foods would mean that people could comply with government health recommendations on fat intake without

having to change their eating habits (Shingfield *et al.*, 2013). This brave new world approach to how we eat is called nutrigenomics. The simpler alternative would be to just eat healthier food!

In addition to the fatty acids discussed there are small amounts of phospholipids and other fats present in milk including fat soluble vitamins.

Minerals and vitamins
Minerals found in cow's milk include sodium, potassium, calcium, magnesium, phosphorus and chloride, zinc, iron (although at extremely low levels), selenium, iodine and trace amounts of copper and manganese (FSA, 2002). Vitamins in cow's milk include retinol, carotene, vitamin E, thiamin, riboflavin, niacin, vitamin B6, vitamin B12, folate, pantothenate, biotin, vitamin C and trace amounts of vitamin D (FSA, 2002). In the US, milk is fortified with additional vitamin D; this has important implications as we shall see later (see Osteoporosis).

Although cow's milk contains all these nutrients it is important to note that these vitamins are contained at very low levels. Furthermore, the mineral content is so out of balance with human biochemistry that it is difficult for us to absorb the optimum amounts required for health.

Fibre
Milk contains no dietary fibre.

The undesirable components of milk and dairy products

Whole milk, cheese, butter and many other dairy products contain high levels of saturated fat, cholesterol and animal protein all of which are not required in the diet and have been linked to a wide range of illnesses and diseases. For example, excess saturated fat and cholesterol in the diet is associated with an increased risk of heart disease and stroke. Cross cultural studies show that as the consumption of saturated fat, cholesterol and animal protein increases from country to country, so does the incidence of the so-called diseases of affluence such as obesity, heart disease, diabetes, osteoporosis and certain cancers. It has been suggested that this is because of genetic differences between different races. However, when people migrate from an area of low incidence of the so-called affluent diseases to an area of high incidence, they soon acquire the same high incidence shared by the population into which they have moved. This correlation must then be attributed, at least in part, to environmental factors such as diet and lifestyle. So if you can increase the risk of disease by changing your diet and lifestyle, it stands to reason that you can reduce the risk of disease by changing your diet and lifestyle. The World Health Organisation (WHO) state that there are major health benefits in eating more fruit and vegetables, as well as nuts and whole grains and moving from saturated animal fats to unsaturated vegetable oil-based fats (WHO, 2003).

In addition to saturated fat, cholesterol and animal protein, a wide range of undesirable components occur in cow's milk and dairy products. The modern dairy cow is prone to both stress and disease. In the UK, cows suffer from a range of infectious diseases including brucellosis, bovine tuberculosis, foot and mouth disease, viral pneumonia and Johne's disease. As a result of an infectious disease a wide range of contaminants can occur in milk. Mastitis (inflammation of the mammary gland) is a widespread condition affecting cattle in the UK in which all or part of the udder suffers from an infection caused by bacteria entering through the teat (Dairy Co, 2013b). Mastitis may be referred to as subclinical (no symptoms) or clinical whereby symptoms include swelling, pain, hardness, milk clots or discoloured milk. The cow responds to the infection by generating white blood cells (somatic cells) which migrate to the affected area in an effort to combat the infection. These cells, along with cellular debris and necrotic (dead) tissue, are a component of pus and are excreted into the milk. Mastitis treatment and control is one of the largest costs to the dairy industry in the UK. Financial losses arise from:

- Milk thrown away due to contamination by medication or being unfit to drink
- A reduction in yields due to illness and any permanent damage to udder tissue
- The extra labour required to tend to mastitic cows
- The costs of veterinary care and medicines
- The cost of reduced longevity due to premature culling

Source: Dairy Co, 2013b.

The number of somatic cells in the milk (the somatic cell count) provides an indication of the level of infection present. These measurements are taken from the milk bulk tank and not from individual cows, so milk from a diseased cow is diluted, especially in larger herds. The somatic cell count usually forms part of a payment structure to farmers with defined thresholds of concentration determining the qualification for bonus payments or penalty charges. Indeed, milk contracts often define several somatic cell count thresholds and any respective bonus for attaining them (Dairy Co 2013c). In most developed dairy industries various regulatory limits are applied to milk for human consumption. In the European Union the somatic cell limit is a maximum of 400,000 cells per ml in bulk milk (Dairy Products (Hygiene) Regulations 1995). **This means that milk containing 400 million pus cells per litre can be sold legally for human consumption. So one teaspoonful of milk could contain up to two million pus cells!** It could be even worse, as concerns have been raised about the efficiency of cell counting techniques (Berry et al., 2003).

Goat's milk is no better. According to the Universities Federation for Animal Welfare (UFAW), 65 per cent of goat milk samples will have a cell count greater than 1,000 million cells per litre (Mowlem, 2011).

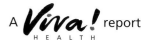

Mastitis effects the quality of milk in many ways; the total protein content is decreased, the amounts of calcium, phosphorus and potassium content are decreased, the taste deteriorates (becomes bitter), and the levels of undesirable components rise. These include enzymes such as plasmin and lipase, and immunoglobulins (Blowey and Edmondson, 2000). Mastitis is treated with antibiotics delivered directly into the udder. These drugs can also end up in the milk, so milk from treated cows must not be marketed until the recommended withholding period has elapsed. Mastitis occurs in around 50 per cent of cows in the UK (Blowey and Edmondson, 2000).

Recent studies show that the value of mammalian milk is not just nutritional but that it contains a variety of factors (biologically active molecules) with additional qualities that have a profound role in the survival and health of the offspring consuming it. These biologically active molecules include enzymes, hormones and growth factors. In 1992, Pennsylvania State University endocrinologist Clark Grosvenor published an extensive review of some of the known bioactive hormones and growth factors found in a typical glass of cow's milk in the US. The list included seven pituitary (an endocrine gland in the brain) hormones, seven steroid hormones, seven hypothalamic (another brain endocrine gland) hormones, eight gastrointestinal peptides (chains of two or more amino acids), six thyroid and parathyroid hormones, 11 growth factors, and nine other biologically active compounds (Grosvenor et al., 1992).

Other biologically important proteins and peptides in milk include immunoglobulins, allergens, enzymes, casomorphins (casein peptide fragments) and cyclic nucleotides (signalling molecules). The concern here is that these signalling molecules that have evolved to direct the rapid growth of the offspring for which they were intended. So, cow's milk, 'designed' to turn a calf into a cow, may initiate inappropriate signalling pathways in the human body that may lead to illnesses and diseases such as cancer.

All milk produced by mammals is a medium for transporting hundreds of different chemical messengers. Human breast milk is a dynamic, multifaceted infant food containing a wide range of nutrients and bioactive factors needed for human infant health and development: macrophages, stem cells, immunoglobulins, cytokines, chemokines, growth factors, hormones, oligosaccharides, glycans and glycosaminoglycans (Ballard and Morrow, 2013). While many studies of human milk composition have been conducted, components of human milk are still being identified. Mammalian milk 'communicates' between the maternal mammary epithelia and the infant's intestinal system directing and educating the immune, metabolic and microflora systems within the infant (German et al., 1992). Indeed, research indicates that many of these molecules survive the environment of the infant's gut and are absorbed into the circulation where they may exert an influence on the infant's immune system, intestinal tract, neuroendocrine system, or take some other effect. This has evolved as a useful mechanism between mothers and infants of the same species, but the effects of bioactive substances in milk taken from one species and consumed by another are largely unknown. The concern is that the bioactive molecules in cow's milk may direct undesirable regulation, growth and differentiation of various tissues in the human infant. Of particular concern for example is the insulin-like growth factor 1 (IGF-1) which occurs naturally in milk and has been linked to several cancers in humans (see IGF-1).

Breast is Best

A substantial body of evidence shows that breastfeeding has important advantages for both infant and mother. Babies receive an important boost to their immune system in the first few days of breastfeeding as important antibodies are passed from the mother to the infant in the colostrum (the fluid expressed before the so-called true milk). These antibodies protect the baby from infection. But that is just the start of it; breastfed babies may have better neurological development than artificially fed infants. They may have better cholesterol and blood pressure levels. More research is needed, but breastfeeding may also provide protection against: multiple sclerosis, acute appendicitis and tonsillectomy. Numerous studies show that the risk of obesity in later life is reduced in people who breastfed as infants (Harder *et al*., 2005; Arenz *et al*., 2004; Owen *et al*., 2005). Women who were breastfed as infants are at lower risk of: breast cancer, ovarian cancer, hip fractures and reduced bone density. Mothers who breastfeed their infants may have a lower risk of rheumatoid arthritis, type 2 diabetes and postnatal

depression (UNICEF, 2013). On the other hand, artificially fed babies are at greater risk of: gastro-intestinal infection, respiratory infections, necrotising enterocolitis, urinary tract infections, ear infections, allergies (eczema and wheezing), type 1 and type 2 diabetes, sudden infant death syndrome and childhood leukaemia (UNICEF, 2013).

UNICEF state that:

> *Formula is not an acceptable substitute for breast milk because formula, at its best, only replaces most of the nutritional components of breast milk: it is just a food, whereas breast milk is a complex living nutritional fluid containing anti-bodies, enzymes, long chain fatty acids and hormones, many of which simply cannot be included in formula. Furthermore, in the first few months, it is hard for the baby's gut to absorb anything other than breast milk. Even one feeding of formula or other foods can cause injuries to the gut, taking weeks for the baby to recover (UNICEF, 2005).*

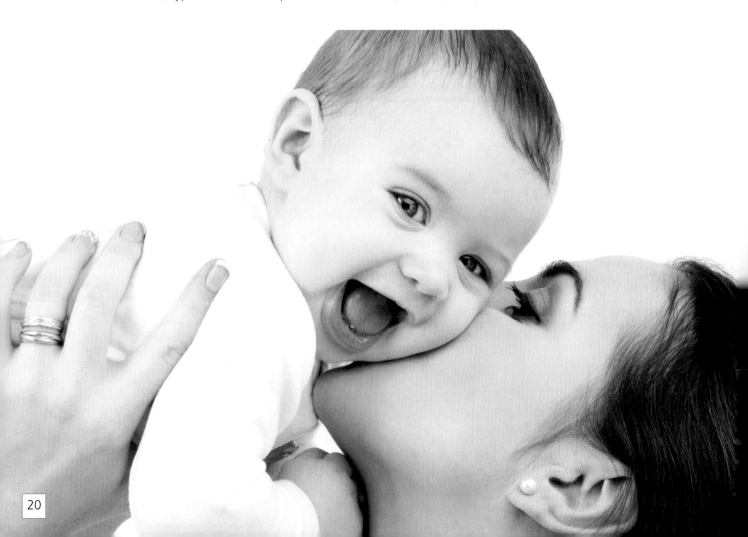

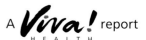

Furthermore, breastfeeding is free. You do not need to wash and sterilise an endless number of bottles. You will not be up in the night mixing and testing the milk to see if it is cool enough; breast milk comes ready mixed at the perfect temperature. The act of breastfeeding is also important for bonding the mother and baby relationship.

In 2013, figures from the Department of Health revealed that the number of new mothers attempting to breastfeed fell in England for the first time since it began collecting the statistics in 2004. The figures showed that 5,700 fewer women initiated breastfeeding with their child in 2012-2013 than did the year before. During this period, 327,048 women (just under half of all maternities) were not breastfeeding their baby at all by the time of their eight week check-up (Royal College of Paediatrics and Health, 2013). This prompted the Royal College of Midwives to express concern over a lack of promotion of breastfeeding under the current Government, which scrapped funding for National Breastfeeding Awareness Week in 2011. The Royal College of Midwives said there is a shortage of 5,000 midwives and criticised the scrapping of infant feeding coordinators, who encouraged breastfeeding in parts of the country with the lowest uptake.

UNICEF states that the major problems are the societal and commercial pressure to stop breastfeeding, including aggressive marketing and promotion by formula producers (UNICEF, 2013a). In addition, many mothers have to return to work soon after giving birth and they face a number of challenges and pressures which often lead them to stop exclusive breastfeeding early. Clearly, mothers (including working mothers) need support, including legislative measures, to enable them to continue breastfeeding. Strategies to promote breastfeeding could confer important and widespread health benefits.

Infant Formula

Some mothers are unable to, or choose not to, breastfeed and in these circumstances infant formula milk is used. Formula milk is designed to meet the nutritional requirements of the infant and must

comply with strict UK and EC legislation which specifies the nutritional composition of the feeds. Soya-based infant formulas provide a safe feeding option for most infants that meet all the nutritional requirements of the infant with none of the detrimental effects associated with the consumption of cow's milk formulas. Under no circumstances should a child under 12 months be given 'normal' cow's, goat's, soya or any other milk that is not specifically formulated for an infant (for a review on the safety of soya see Appendix I).

Milk in Schools

In 1924, local education authorities (LEAs) in the UK were permitted to provide children with free milk. This was the start of the movement to introduce milk to school-aged children that would continue to this day. In 2005, in a paper published in the *Economic History Review*, Dr Peter Atkins of Durham University reviewed the motivations behind the introduction of cow's milk in schools during the first half of the twentieth century (Atkins, 2005). Atkins stated that the nutritional benefits of school milk were debatable, possibly even negative in those areas where it replaced other foods, but noted that the dairy industry did well, creating new markets at a time of depression (Atkins, 2005).

In 1946, the School Milk Act provided free milk to all school children. A third of a pint of milk was provided to all children under the age of 18 years until 1968 when Harold Wilson's Government withdrew free milk from secondary schools. This policy was extended in 1971 when Margaret Thatcher (then secretary of state for education) withdrew free school milk from children over seven. This was an economic decision, not one based on a nutritional assessment of the value of milk, and for this she earned the nickname 'Thatcher, Thatcher, milk snatcher' – although many children were delighted at not having to drink the warm sickly odorous milk at school anymore!

The school milk scheme was introduced in 1977 by the European Union (EU) to encourage the consumption of milk in schools. The scheme required member states to make subsidised milk available to primary and nursery schools wishing to take part, but participation was entirely a matter for the school or LEA. The European Commission had originally indicated that it wished to abolish the subsidy because the scheme was not providing value for money. The UK did not accept these conclusions and fought hard to retain the scheme. A compromise was secured whereby in 2001 the subsidy rate was reduced from 95 to 75 per cent. The UK Government topped up the subsidy to its original level in England, up to a maximum total expenditure of £1.5 million each year. In the academic year 2003 to 2004, around one million school children in England drank 34.9 million litres of subsidised milk at a cost of around £7 million.

The move to increase milk consumption in schools gathered momentum; the School Milk Project, was set up in 1998 by the Women's Food and Farming Union, aiming to increase the uptake of milk in primary schools. It received funding from the Milk Development Council (MDC) which was established following the re-organisation of the milk industry in 1994. The MDC was funded by a statutory levy on all milk sold off farms in Great Britain; the annual income from the levy was over £7 million. Primarily the MDC funded research and development into milk production methods, it also funded the School Milk Project which employed 'facilitators' to promote the uptake of school milk through direct contact with LEAs, schools and dairy suppliers.

The charity Milk For Schools (MFS) was founded in 1994. Set up to educate the public in the field of school based nutrition, MFS is a registered member of the United Nations Food and Agriculture Organisation (UNFAO) School Milk Network, which initiated the first World School Milk Day on 27th September 2000. In October 2004 Dairy UK was established as a cross-industry body representing processors and distributors of liquid milk and dairy products, as well as milk producer co-operatives. In 2005 the European Union (EU) and Dairy UK joined forces with the MDC to promote milk consumption in primary schools. Schools were targeted with 'Teacher's Guides to Health and Fitness' and School Milk Week

commenced on 10th October 2005. Previous school milk weeks have generated over 6,000 new school milk drinkers or as Dairy UK put it "over one million new serving opportunities per annum".

In 2008, the MDC was replaced by DairyCo following a fundamental review of agricultural levy boards by Defra. The five existing levy boards (including the MDC) were replaced by one statutory levy board, the Agriculture and Horticulture Development Board (AHDB). Its statutory purpose is to improve UK farm business efficiency and competitiveness. In 2010 DairyCo conducted a full review of in school activities and re-launched its Schools and Education programme in January 2011 which replaced The School Milk Project. DairyCo works alongside the British Nutrition Foundation (another industry-funded body) to promote milk in schools using a range of tools including web-based education resources promoting dairy products. To this end, DairyCo offers free resources and advice to local authorities and schools about milk production and dairy farming and how to introduce or increase milk provision in their schools.

This sophisticated and aggressive marketing is of real value to the dairy industry in establishing milk as a 'normal' commodity for regular family consumption now and in the future. The policy of introducing school milk begs the question, are the dairy industry nurturing our children? Or simply nurturing a future loyal adult consumer base?

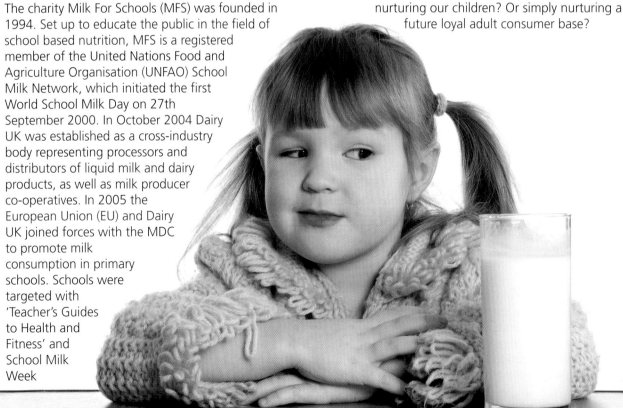

Part two:
Dairy Consumption and Health

The suggestion that the consumption of cow's milk can lead to a wide range of health problems, illnesses and diseases strikes at the core of many people's thinking. How can such a natural food be unhealthy? Well the answer lies in the fact that milk is not a natural drink for adults. Furthermore, cow's milk is not a natural drink for humans. In nature, milk is consumed from a mother up until weaning, which is when the mother normally stops producing milk. Consuming milk from a pregnant mother is not the normal course of events. Furthermore, in nature, mammals consume the milk of their own species, not that of another. In a commentary published in the *Journal of the American Academy of Dermatology*, New Hampshire dermatologist Dr F.W. Danby states that the human consumption of large volumes of another species' milk, especially when that milk comes from pregnant cows during the human's normally post-weaned years, is essentially unnatural (Danby, 2005).

As previously stated, cow's milk is designed to help a small calf grow into a big cow in less than a year. In order to sustain this rapid physical growth, the composition of cow's milk has evolved to contain the specific types of nutrients required, at the specific levels required. These are not necessarily natural or healthy for humans. For example, whole milk and certain dairy products such as butter and cheese, contain considerable amounts of saturated fat, cholesterol and animal protein, the detrimental health effects of which are now well-documented. In addition to this, the vitamin and mineral content of cow's milk is not well-suited to human requirements, especially those of the human infant. To meet the rapid skeletal growth requirements of a calf, cow's milk contains four times the amount of calcium as human milk. This does not mean that cow's milk is a good source of calcium for the human infant, far from it; this level of calcium coupled to the high levels of other minerals in cow's milk represents what is called a high renal solute load which means that the young human infant's kidneys cannot cope with 'off the shelf' cow's milk.

In addition to the unsuitable nutritional composition of cow's milk, there are many other reasons why cow's milk and dairy products are not natural foods for humans, for example, the increasing body of evidence linking bioactive molecules in milk (hormones and growth factors) to disease. While the dairy industry would have us believe that milk is an essential part of the diet, much of the research used to promote this view is industry-sponsored.

Furthermore, given that around 70 per cent of people in the world do not drink milk, just how essential can it be? The list of illnesses and diseases associated with the consumption of milk and dairy products is quite extensive. These health problems tend to occur at levels that relate directly to how much milk is drunk in a particular region or country. Furthermore, as milk consumption spreads to areas where previously it was not drunk, these diseases follow. Some of these problems are discussed in detail below.

Acne

Acne is a skin condition that affects many teenagers and in a small number of cases it may occur in adulthood. About 80 per cent of people between the ages of 11 and 30 will be affected by acne. It is most common between the ages of 14 and 17 in girls, and between 16 and 19 in boys. Acne can continue into adult life; about five per cent of women and one per cent of men have acne over the age of 25 (NHS Choices, 2012a).

Acne can cause physical scarring but it can also cause distress, anxiety and depression in some sufferers who report feeling suicidal because of bullying or lack of self-confidence.

Acne is caused by a combination of factors. Hormonal changes can increase the secretion of an oily substance called sebum from the skin's sebaceous glands which are frequently located adjacent to hair follicles. If skin cells build up and block the opening of hair follicles, subsequent clogging of the sebaceous gland can contribute further to the development of acne. The problem is often made even worse by the colonisation of the skin by the bacterium *Propionibacterium acnes* which can become trapped in the hair follicles. Inflammation then may lead to the eruption of large pus-filled spots characteristic of acne. Despite the wholesale dismissal of diet as a potential environmental factor underlying the development of acne, a large body of evidence now exists that demonstrates how certain foods and food substances (especially cow's milk) may adversely influence hormones and cytokines that influence the causes of acne (Cordain, 2005).

A large-scale study from Harvard's School of Public Health linked the intake of milk during adolescence with the incidence of acne in 47,355 nurses who

23

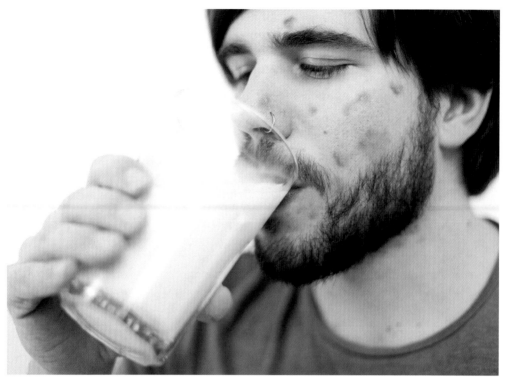

completed questionnaires on high school diet and teenage acne (Adebamowo *et al.*, 2005). The link between teenage acne and milk consumption was strongest for skimmed milk, so it would seem that the saturated fat content of milk is not the causal factor. The authors hypothesised that the hormonal content of milk may be responsible for causing acne in teenagers. Cow's milk contains the hormones oestrogen and progesterone along with certain hormone precursors (androstenedione, dehydroepiandrosterone-sulphate, and 5 -reduced steroids like 5 -androstanedione, 5 -pregnanedione and dihydrotestosterone), some of which have been implicated in the development of acne.

The levels of these hormones in cow's milk vary depending on whether the cow is pregnant or not, and if so at what stage of the pregnancy she is. At least two-thirds of cow's milk in the UK is taken from pregnant cows (Danby, 2005). The same team of researchers have produced two subsequent articles based on the nurses' sons and daughters. In these groups too, a positive association was observed between dairy products (particularly skimmed milk) and acne (Adebamowo *et al.*, 2006; Adebamowo *et al.*, 2008). Again, this suggests that it is some component in cow's milk other than saturated fat that causes acne.

Body builders who use steroid hormones to stimulate muscle growth and strength are more prone to acne as many of the side effects of steroids are manifested in the skin. This also applies to athletes who use whey-based supplements for weight gain as these protein powders increase IGF-1 and insulin levels, both of which are linked to acne. A number of recent studies have revealed a link between whey protein and acne. One case study showed that healthy male adults developed acne after the consumption of whey protein (Simonart, 2012). Another found that benzoyl peroxide cream or oral antibiotics had little effect on treating the serious acne affecting five young men who used whey supplements. However, when they stopped using whey, their acne became less severe and was treatable (Silverberg, 2012). The author of this study

recommends that use of whey protein supplements should be screened for when taking history from teenage males suffering with acne.

Milk also contains many bioactive molecules that act on the sebaceous glands and hair follicles (such as glucocorticoids, IGF-1, transforming growth factor-β (TGF-β), neutral thyrotropin-releasing hormone-like peptides and opiate-like compounds), some of which survive pasteurisation. The bioavailability of the factors involved may be altered during pasteurisation. In other words, heat-induced changes in the shape or structure of the molecule may alter the way it behaves in the body and, until we know more, it is difficult to say exactly what role these bioactive molecules play in causing acne and other health problems. However, the current literature leaves no room for doubt that dairy products increase the risk of acne. In summary, to help eliminate or avoid acne, eat more fruit and vegetables and stay away from cow's milk and dairy products.

Allergies

The body's immune system has to constantly discriminate between many different unfamiliar molecules, some of which may be toxic substances while others are harmless components of food. An allergy results from an inappropriate immune response to such a substance (or allergen) such as dust, pollen or a component of food. An allergic reaction occurs as the body attempts to launch an attack against the foreign 'invader' perceived to be a threat to health. In such an attack, the body releases a substance called histamine, which dilates and increases the permeability of the small blood vessels. This results in a range of symptoms including local inflammation, sneezing, runny nose, itchy eyes and

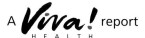
so on. These types of reactions may give rise to the so-called classic allergies: asthma, eczema, hay fever and urticaria (skin rash). These responses are called anaphylactic reactions and they vary widely in their severity. The most severe type of reaction (anaphylactic shock) may involve difficulty in breathing, a drop in blood pressure and ultimately heart failure and death.

Initial sensitisation to the allergen precedes an allergic reaction and this first exposure may not generate any perceivable symptoms. In fact initial sensitisation may result not from the direct exposure to an allergen but from exposure to dietary allergens during breastfeeding. Evidence suggests that this process, known as atopic sensitisation, can occur in exclusively breastfed infants whose mother's breast milk contains dietary allergens. For example, a Finnish study reported that a maternal diet rich in saturated fat during breastfeeding might be a risk factor underlying the later development of allergies (Hoppu *et al.*, 2000). The same research group later reported that breast milk rich in saturated fat and low in omega-3 fatty acids might be a risk factor for eczema (Hoppu *et al.*, 2005). While numerous studies now show that breastfeeding can protect against the development of allergies, and the majority of studies are strongly in favour of breastfeeding, it may be prudent to avoid suspected allergens in the diet while breastfeeding especially if allergies such as asthma, eczema and hay fever run in the family.

Allergies are now so common in the UK, affecting around one in three people, that the increasing occurrence is referred to by some as an epidemic (Royal College of Physicians, 2003). The UK is one of the top countries in the world for the highest incidence of allergy, especially asthma. Millions of adults in the UK are affected by at least one allergy and numbers continue to rise (Allergy UK, 2013). Each year the number of allergy sufferers increases by five per cent, half of all affected being children, and by 2015, 50 per cent Europeans will suffer from an allergy (EFA, 2011).

Food allergy is increasingly widespread and the most common of these is cow's milk allergy, affecting around two per cent of all infants under the age of one. Symptoms include excessive mucus production resulting in a runny nose and blocked ears. More serious symptoms include asthma, eczema, colic, diarrhoea and vomiting.

Asthma

Asthma is a chronic, inflammatory lung disease characterised by recurrent breathing problems. Asthma is a common condition in the UK; 5.4 million people are currently receiving treatment for asthma (NHS Choices, 2012b). That is one in every 12 adults and one in every 11 children. The number of children with asthma has risen steeply since the 1970s when just one in 50 children had asthma. Asthma prevalence is thought to have plateaued since the late 1990s, although the UK still has some of the highest rates in Europe and on average three people a day die from asthma (Asthma UK, 2013).

During an asthma attack, the lining of the airways becomes inflamed and the airways become narrower causing the characteristic symptoms of asthma: coughing, wheezing, difficulty in breathing and tightness across the chest. Asthma can start at any age and the causes are thought to include a combination of factors including a genetic predisposition (asthma in the family), diet and environmental triggers such as cigarette smoke, chemicals and dust mites.

As stated previously, allergies tend to run in families, so asthma, eczema or hay fever in some family members may increase the risk of others developing the same or another allergy. But a genetic predisposition is not the only cause, as stated asthma is caused by a combination of factors. In the past, the rise in childhood asthma has been attributed to an increase in air pollution. However, this seems unlikely as many of the most polluted countries in the world, such as China, have low rates of asthma, whereas countries with very good air quality, such as New Zealand, have high rates of asthma (ISAAC, 1998). The 'hygiene hypothesis' has gained popularity as a causal factor for the increase in asthma. This hypothesis blames the increasing asthma rates on the extreme levels of cleanliness found in many homes. Increased hygiene means that our immune systems are being challenged less and less. It has been suggested that this causes us to overreact to allergens such as dust mites.

Food allergy is frequently underestimated in association with asthma despite the fact that food allergy and asthma frequently co-exist. Children with food allergy are more than two to four times as likely to have other atopic conditions such as asthma, eczema or respiratory allergy compared to children without food allergies (Kewalramani and Bollinger, 2010). Furthermore, food allergy has been shown to trigger or exacerbate broncho-obstruction in two to 8.5 per cent of children with asthma (Baena-Cagnani and Teijeiro, 2001). Food allergies may be responsible for around five per cent of all asthma cases (James *et al.*, 1994) and as cow's milk is a primary cause of food allergies, it may therefore be useful to consider the possibility of cow's milk allergy in the treatment of asthma.

Eczema

Eczema (also known as atopic dermatitis) is a condition that causes the skin to become itchy, red, dry and cracked. It is a long-term, chronic condition.

Eczema can vary in severity and most people are only mildly affected but severe symptoms can include cracked, sore and bleeding skin. Severe eczema can have a significant impact on daily life. The number of people diagnosed with atopic eczema has increased in recent years and currently, about one in five children and one in 12 adults in the UK have eczema (NHS Choices, 2012b; National Eczema Society 2013).

Cow's milk allergy is a risk factor for many allergic conditions including asthma and eczema (Saarinen, 2005). There is an increasing amount of interest in the role of the diet in the development of eczema. In recent years, the links between certain foods and eczema has become better understood. Eczema can be caused by several environmental factors including dust mites, grasses and pollens, stress and certain foods. Eczema usually starts when a baby is around six months old and in about 10 per cent of cases it is triggered by foods including milk, eggs, citrus fruit, chocolate, peanuts and colourings (NHS Choices, 2013c). The most common food triggers are cow's milk and eggs, but many other foods including soya, wheat, fish and nuts can act as triggers (National Eczema Society 2013a). So, when treating eczema, cow's milk allergy should be considered.

Hay fever

Hay fever (seasonal allergic rhinitis) is an allergic reaction to grass or hay pollens. A minority of cases may be caused by later flowering weeds or fungal spores, and some research suggests pollution can worsen symptoms. In response to exposure to pollen, the immune system releases histamine which gives rise to a range of symptoms including a runny nose, sneezing and itchy eyes and throat. Hay fever is often regarded as a trivial problem but it can severely affect people's quality of life, disturbing sleep, impairing daytime concentration, it causes people to miss work or school and has been shown to affect school exam results (Allergy UK, 2012).

Hay fever is one of the most common allergic conditions that affects up to one in five people at some point in their life. Hay fever is more likely if there is a family history of allergies, particularly asthma or eczema (NHS Choices, 2011). Some evidence suggests that altering the diet can help some people with asthma and allergic rhinitis (Ogle and Bullock, 1980). However, the effects of diet on hay fever symptoms have not yet been well studied. As cow's milk allergy is linked to other allergic reactions (see above) it may be sensible to consider avoiding all dairy in order to combat hay fever symptoms.

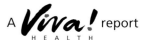

Gastrointestinal bleeding

As stated above, cow's milk-induced gastrointestinal bleeding as an allergic response is a well-recognised cause of rectal bleeding in infancy (Willetts *et al.*, 1999). One of the main causes of gastrointestinal bleeding is dietary protein allergy, the most common cause of which is cow's milk protein (casein). Gastrointestinal bleeding from cow's milk allergy often occurs in such small quantities that the blood loss is not detected visually, but over prolonged time these losses can cause iron-deficiency anaemia in children. Intestinal blood loss associated with cow's milk consumption during infancy affects about 40 per cent of otherwise healthy infants (Ziegler *et al.*, 2011). In one trial of 52 infants, 31 of whom had been breastfed, and 21 fed formulas up to the age of 168 days of age, the introduction of cow's milk (rather than formula milk) was associated with an increased blood loss from the intestinal tract and a nutritionally important loss of iron (Ziegler *et al.*, 1990).

Frank Oski, former paediatrics director at Johns Hopkins School of Medicine, estimates that half the iron-deficiency in infants in the US results from cow's milk-induced gastrointestinal bleeding (Oski, 1996). This represents a staggering figure since more than 15 per cent of US infants under the age of two suffer from iron-deficiency anaemia.

The only reliable treatment for cow's milk allergy is to avoid all cow's milk and dairy products including: milk, milk powder, milk drinks, cheese, butter, margarine, yogurt, cream and ice cream. Also products with hidden milk content should be avoided. Food labels that list any of the following ingredients also contain some cow's milk or products in them: casein, caseinates, hydrolysed casein, skimmed milk, skimmed milk powder, milk solids, non-fat milk, whey, whey syrup sweetener, milk sugar solids. These ingredients can be difficult to avoid as they are commonly used in the production of bread, processed cereals, instant soups, margarine, salad dressings, sweets, cake mix and even crisps. It can seem a daunting prospect having to read the ingredients labels but most supermarkets now produce 'free-from' lists of products and many supermarkets also have their own-label free-from range. There are even iPhone apps available now to help you identify ingredients by scanning the product bar code. Soya ice creams, spreads and yoghurts and dairy-free cheeses are just some examples. Calcium-enriched soya, rice and oat milks can be used as alternatives to cow's milk. (For other gastrointestinal problems associated with cow's milk see Lactose intolerance.)

Arthritis

Millions of people in the UK experience some form of musculoskeletal problem each year. Around nine million people seek help from their GP each year, of these, more than two million have osteoarthritis and more than 350,000 have rheumatoid arthritis. About 15,000 children and adolescents suffer from juvenile forms of arthritis (Arthritis Research UK, 2013).

Osteoarthritis, the most common form of arthritis in the UK, affects an estimated 8.5 million people and often develops in people who are over 50 years of age (NHS Choices, 2012d). Osteoarthritis is a degenerative disease where articular cartilage gradually becomes thinner as its renewal does not keep pace with its breakdown. Eventually the bony articular surfaces come into contact and the bones begin to degenerate. Osteoarthritis can develop after an injury to a joint; this can happen months or even years after the injury. The most frequently affected joints are in the hands, knees, feet, hips and spine.

The next most common type of arthritis is rheumatoid arthritis, a chronic inflammatory disease of the joints. In the UK, rheumatoid arthritis affects around 400,000 people and often starts in people between the ages of 40 and 50 years old. Women are three times more likely to be affected by the condition than men. (NHS Choices, 2012d). Rheumatoid arthritis is a chronic condition characterised by hot painful swelling in the joints. In many diseases inflammation can help towards healing but in rheumatoid arthritis it tends to cause damage. For some people the pain and discomfort caused by this condition has a serious impact on their lives. Rheumatoid arthritis is thought to be an autoimmune disease, caused by a fault in the immune system that causes the body to attack its own tissues. This condition usually starts in the wrists, hands and feet but can spread to other joints in the body.

Other forms of arthritis include: ankylosing spondylitis, cervical spondylitis, fibromyalgia, lupus, gout, psoriatic arthritis, reactive arthritis, secondary arthritis and polymyalgia rheumatica (NHS Choices, 2012d). In the UK, about 12,000 children under 16 years of age have arthritis. Most types of childhood arthritis are referred to as juvenile idiopathic arthritis and although the exact causes are unknown, the symptoms often improve as a child gets older, allowing them to lead a normal life (NHS Choices, 2012d).

There has been a general reluctance to acknowledge the links between diet and arthritis with a tendency to dismiss anecdotal evidence. However, studies show that people who eat a lot of red meat may have a higher risk of developing inflammatory types of arthritis. It has also been suggested that dairy may trigger an inappropriate autoimmune response in some people who may then go on to develop rheumatoid arthritis via a mechanism called molecular mimicry. This may occur when antibodies react to a protein in cow's milk called bovine serum albumin, mistaking it for an antigen or foreign protein.

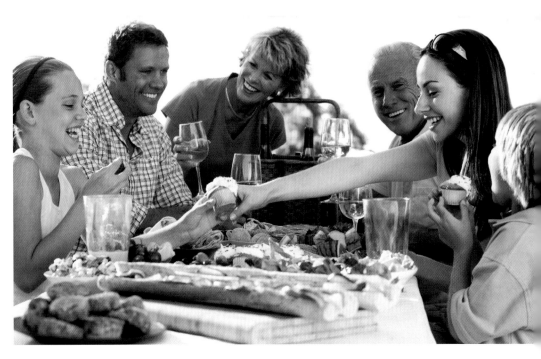

Some studies have looked at the effects of a vegan diet on the symptoms of arthritis. A single-blind dietary intervention study investigated the effects of a very low-fat, vegan diet on patients with rheumatoid arthritis (McDougall *et al.*, 2002). This study evaluated the influence of a four-week, low-fat, vegan diet on 24 people with rheumatoid arthritis. The results showed a significant decrease in symptoms. The degree of pain dramatically reduced; limitation in ability to function improved, joint tenderness and joint swelling significantly decreased. The severity of morning stiffness improved, the only thing not to improve was the duration of the morning stiffness. The researchers concluded that patients with moderate-to-severe rheumatoid arthritis, who switch to a very low-fat, vegan diet can experience significant reductions in their symptoms.

It is now accepted that the Mediterranean diet can help people with arthritis as well as a number of other conditions. This diet includes plenty of fruit and vegetables, fish, grains and pulses and a moderate amount of red meat. Foods rich in omega-3 are believed to have an anti-inflammatory effect, which may reduce the pain associated with inflamed joints. Omega-3 is found in nuts and seeds (particularly linseed or flax seed) and is regularly used to fortify margarines. (It is also found in oily fish but oily fish also contains PCBs, dioxins and other toxins that are best

avoided by opting for plant-based sources of omega-3s.) It is important for people with arthritis to maintain a healthy well-balanced diet. Arthritis Care (the UK's largest voluntary organisation working with and for people with arthritis) suggest a diet high in fruit, vegetables, starch and fibre and low in fatty foods, salt and added sugars can help (Arthritis Care, 2011).

Some research suggests a high intake of fruit and vegetables may prevent or slow down osteoarthritis. Sulforaphane, a chemical found in vegetables such as broccoli, has been reported to have anti-inflammatory properties, may protect against a form of inflammatory arthritis and reduce the production of enzymes that contribute to the breakdown of cartilage. Indeed a recent study from the University of East Anglia looked at human cartilage cells treated with cytokines and found that sulforaphane reduced the production of enzymes involved in cartilage damage (Davidson *et al.*, 2013). This suggests that sulforaphane could help reduce cartilage damage and prevent or slow the progression of arthritis. Most people could benefit from eating more fruit and vegetables, complex carbohydrates, fibre, vitamins and minerals and less sugar and saturated fat.

If you suffer from arthritis it is important to keep as healthy as possible by ensuring that the diet provides

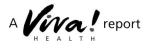

all the important nutrients including minerals such as calcium and iron. Some people are concerned that their calcium intake may drop if they cut out dairy foods. Arthritis Care state that dairy products are not the only sources of calcium and that you can reach the recommended daily amount by eating a variety of calcium-rich foods (Arthritis Care, 2010). They list several non-dairy sources of calcium including watercress, tofu, figs, Brazil nuts, bread and baked beans. Be careful not to have too much salt or caffeine as excessive quantities of these can reduce the body's ability to absorb or retain calcium.

Others are worried about iron, particularly people who have recently stopped eating red meat. This should not be a concern as vegetarians and vegans are no more likely to become iron deficient than meat-eaters. Indeed one of the largest studies of vegetarians and vegans in the world (the EPIC Oxford cohort study) looked at over 33,883 meat-eaters, 18,840 vegetarians and 2,596 vegans and found that the vegans had the highest intake of iron, followed by the vegetarians then the meat-eaters (Davey *et al.*, 2003). It should be stressed that milk and milk products are an extremely poor source of iron, whereas pulses, dried fruits and dark leafy vegetables are good sources.

The Arthritis Research Campaign (now Arthritis Research UK) founded in 1936, raises funds to promote medical research into the cause, treatment and cure of arthritic conditions. They have produced dietary guidelines for people with arthritis and they suggest that one of the most important links between diet and arthritis is being overweight. The extra burden on the joints can make symptoms considerably worse. Losing weight can have a dramatic effect in improving the condition. In order to lose weight, you need to use more energy than you consume in the diet. Research shows that vegetarians and vegans weigh less than meat-eaters and Arthritis Research UK suggests that vegetarian diets have been shown to be helpful in the long term for some people with rheumatoid arthritis. A vegan diet, which doesn't include any meat, fish or other animal products, may also be helpful, possibly because of the types of polyunsaturated fatty acids included in the diet (Arthritis Research UK, 2013a). Cutting down on sugar and taking regular (even gentle) exercise will help control weight as well.

Saturated fats are the most important kind of fat to cut down on. The body does not require saturated fats and they may aggravate arthritis whereas

essential fatty acids (EFAs) have been shown to help some people with arthritis. These polyunsaturated fatty acids are divided into two main groups: omega-3 and omega-6. Omega-3 fatty acids are thought to be of most benefit in inflammatory arthritis (Arthritis Research UK, 2013a).

When trying to lose weight, it is important to maintain a good intake of vitamins and minerals. This means consuming plenty of fruit and vegetables. A healthy balanced diet containing plenty of fruit and vegetables, pulses and whole grain carbohydrate foods (such as wholemeal bread, brown rice and whole wheat pasta) provides a good supply of vitamins, minerals and fibre. A diet lacking in fruit and vegetables, and containing processed carbohydrates (such as white bread, white rice and white pasta) does not provide such a good source of these essential nutrients and can have a deleterious effect on health. Whereas a good diet may help even if strong drugs are being taken to treat arthritis.

The subject of food allergy and arthritis is quite controversial. However, research has shown that, in some people, rheumatoid arthritis can be made worse by certain foods including milk products and food colouring (Laar and Korst, 1992). In 2001, Swedish researchers reported that nine out of 22 patients with rheumatoid arthritis showed significant improvements in their condition compared to one patient out of 25 after following a gluten-free, vegan diet (Hafstrom *et al.*, 2001). Of course it is difficult to say whether eliminating milk was the reason these patients improved as they eliminated all animal foods and gluten from the diet. However, this work provides evidence that dietary modification can benefit arthritis patients. Diet is not the only factor to cause and aggravate rheumatoid arthritis, nor is a vegan diet the only way to reduce or eliminate the pain and damage caused by this disease. However, research shows that a low fat vegan diet can be a powerful and positive, drug free way of limiting the painful symptoms caused by this disease.

Bovine Somatotrophin (BST)

In cows, milk production is influenced by the complex interaction of a range of hormones. Bovine somatotrophin (BST) is a natural growth hormone that occurs in cattle and controls the amount of milk that they produce. In 1994 Monsanto began marketing a synthetic version of BST, known as recombinant BST (rBST), which was sold as Posilac and fast became the largest selling dairy animal pharmaceutical product in the US. In 2008, Monsanto sold the Posilac business to Eli Lilly and Company for $300 million. From 2000-2005 the USDA National Agricultural Statistics Service survey of dairy producers found that about 17 per cent of dairy milk producers used rBST. Injecting dairy cows with rBST alters the metabolism to increase milk production by up to 15 per cent. Monsanto claims that this 'allows' the cow to produce more milk. They also argue that the increased production lowers the cost of milk, making it more affordable, and the number of cows needed to keep current milk production levels is decreased thus saving natural recourses (Monsanto, 2009).

However, there is a cost associated with the use of rBST; its use is associated with severe welfare problems, for example increasing the incidence of lameness and mastitis. While the US Food and Drug Administration (FDA) permit the use of rBST, for reasons of animal health and welfare, the use of rBST in the EU was prohibited in 2000. Indeed Canada, Japan and many other countries have also banned the use of rBST because of its effects on animal health and welfare. However, there are no restrictions on the import of rBST dairy products to the UK, or any requirement to label them.

The Government's Veterinary Medicines Directorate does not carry out any testing of imported milk for rBST (Defra, 2013). Furthermore, Defra confirmed in correspondence with the Viva!Health, that since the EU is a single market once a product has entered, if it is transported on to another country within the EU, then the origin of the product will be the EU country rather than the originating country (Defra, 2013). Over the last decade imports of dairy foods have fallen from around 6,000 tonnes (mainly ice cream) per year to around 1,000. There was a steep rise in 2007 when nearly 4,000 tonnes were imported, and in the last year imports of yoghurt have increased significantly (Defra, 2013a). Although these figures have declined, they still remain a concern, especially as the consumer has a limited chance of discriminating against imports from the US. The sensible option is to avoid all dairy products.

Concern has been expressed over several health issues associated with the use of rBST. The increased incidence of lameness and mastitis in rBST-treated cows inevitably leads to an increased use of antibiotics to treat these and other infections. Because of their efficacy in treating and preventing disease and the fact that they can promote growth in some animals when used at sub-therapeutic levels, antibiotics have been widely used for many years. Over half of the antibiotics that are produced in the US are used for agricultural purposes (Mellon et al., 2001).

Antibiotic use is known to promote the development of antibiotic resistance. Thus the widespread use of these drugs has contributed to the high frequency of resistant bacteria in the intestinal flora of farmed animals (Lipsitch et al., 2002). This raises concerns about the development of antibiotic resistant infections in humans. A study in the New England Journal of Medicine in 2000 reported that the emergence of antibiotic-resistant strains of Salmonella is associated with the use of antibiotics in cattle. This study described how a new antibiotic-resistant strain of Salmonella was isolated from a 12-year-old boy admitted to hospital with abdominal pain, vomiting and diarrhoea. The boy lived on a ranch in Nebraska and subsequent investigation revealed the presence of the identical strain of bacteria, resistant to the antibiotic ceftriaxone, among cattle on his family's ranch and nearby ranches that had suffered outbreaks of salmonellosis. The cattle had been treated with ceftriaxone. This evidence suggests that the boy's gastrointestinal infection was acquired from cattle (Fey et al., 2000).

The use of antibiotics in animals is so widespread now that it may exceed their use in human medicine. As stated, drug-resistance in bacteria is driven by this selective pressure and can spread to humans either by the food supply (meat, fish, eggs and dairy products), direct contact with animals or more indirectly through environmental pathways (da Costa et al., 2013). This may shorten the time that these valuable antimicrobial agents will be available for effective treatment of infections in humans (Hammerum and Heuer, 2009). The obvious concern here is that the widespread use of antibiotics in cattle can lead to an increase in antibiotic-resistant strains that may subsequently transmit to humans. This is a public health concern and the question must be asked: how much evidence of harm do we need

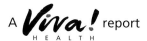

before we much further restrict the use of antibiotics in farm animals?

Milk production increases in cows treated with rBST because it promotes the production of the naturally occurring growth hormone insulin-like growth factor 1 (IGF-1) which then stimulates the glands in the cow's udders to produce more milk. Research shows that rBST use on dairy cows can substantially increase the levels of IGF-1 in their milk (Prosser *et al.*, 1989). IGF-1 in milk is not denatured (inactivated) by pasteurisation. This raises concerns about the potential biological action of IGF-1 from cow's milk in humans especially because IGF-1 from cows is identical to human IGF-1. Professor Samuel Epstein, an international leading authority on the causes and prevention of cancer, warns that converging lines of evidence incriminate IGF-1 in rBST milk as a potential risk factor for both breast and gastrointestinal cancers (Epstein, 1996). However, the extent to which intact, active IGF-1 is absorbed through the human digestive tract remains uncertain (see IGF-1).

So why should this concern us if we do not allow the use of rBST in the UK? Well in terms of human health, the concern is that milk and milk products imported from countries that permit the use of rBST may lead to the consumption of foods that promote increased levels of IGF-1 in humans. In 1999, the minister of state, Baroness Hayman, referred to a report from the Veterinary Products Committee (VPC) which stated that while the use of rBST does not increase the level of BST found naturally in cow's milk, there is a two-to-five fold increase the level of IGF-1 in the milk, which she acknowledged may be implicated in the occurrence of colonic cancer. However, Hayman reiterated the VPC's view that the risk to human health was likely to be extremely small. Hayman also suggested that just 0.3 per cent of total milk and milk products imported into the UK come from the US where rBST is authorised for use (UK Parliament, 1999). While it is not proven that milk produced using rBST increases IGF-1 levels and the risk of cancer in humans, you can avoid these potential risks by avoiding all dairy products.

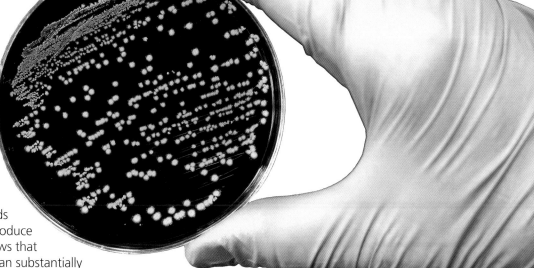

Cancer

More than one in three people in the UK will develop some form of cancer during their lifetime (NHS Choices, 2012u). Around 325,000 people were diagnosed with cancer in 2010 in the UK, that's around 890 people every day. Cancer causes more than one in four of all deaths in the UK. In 2010 around 430 people died from cancer every day; that is one person every four minutes (Cancer Research UK, 2013). The four most common cancers in the UK are breast, prostate, lung and colorectal (bowel) cancer. The data shows that while incidence rates have increased over previous years, mortality rates have fallen. So more people are getting cancer, but less are dying from it. The net result is that mortality from cancer over the last 50 years has remained fairly constant. This is very worrying when you consider the vast improvement in both cancer diagnosis techniques and cancer treatment methods. It means that as even more people are getting cancer, the medical profession are running, just to stand still. It is predicted that by 2020 almost one in two people (47 per cent) will get cancer in their lifetime (Macmillan Cancer Support, 2013). This poses a huge challenge for the NHS and for society.

Up to 40 per cent of cancers in the UK could be prevented by lifestyle changes (Parkin *et al.*, 2010). Most people now recognise that smoking is the biggest single preventable risk factor for cancer. Lung cancer is the UK's biggest cancer killer, causing one in four of all deaths from cancer. Nearly 35,000 people die from lung cancer in the UK every year (NHS Choices, 2013a). Smoking also increases the risk of many other types of cancer, including cancers of the: mouth, pharynx (behind the nose), larynx (voice box), oesophagus, stomach, pancreas, liver, cervix, kidney and bladder. Stopping smoking, even when middle-aged, can dramatically reduce the risk of developing cancer.

However, it is less well known that a poor diet is the second largest preventable risk factor for cancer, coming close behind smoking. Research shows that nutrition plays a major role in cancer (Donaldson, 2004). Indeed a poor diet may be responsible for up to a third of all cancer deaths. Evidence from migration studies from the 1980's shows that plant-based diets can protect against cancer, while typical Western diets, rich in animal foods, sugar and highly processed food products, can increase the risk. Indeed, a significant body of evidence now shows that a plant-based diet, containing less saturated animal fats, cholesterol, animal protein, sugar, salt and processed foods can lower the risk of some cancers and that a diet rich in saturated animal fats, cholesterol, animal protein, sugar, salt and processed foods can increase the risk of certain cancers. Diet has now been linked to numerous types of cancer including cancer of the: bowel, stomach, breast, lung, prostate, pancreas, oesophagus and bladder (Cancer Research UK, 2011).

The link between red and processed meat and cancer is now well-established. In 2007, a review by a team of experts convened by the World Cancer Research Fund (WCRF) and the American Institute for Cancer Research (AICR) concluded that red and processed meats increase the risk of some cancers and that diets rich in plant foods decrease the risk of many types of cancer (WCRF/AICR, 2007). They

specified the beneficial effects of fibre, fruits, vegetables, beans, peas and pulses (including soya foods) and whole grains Their recommendation was as follows. To reduce your cancer risk, eat no more than 500 grams (cooked weight) per week of red meat, like beef, pork and lamb, and avoid processed meats such as ham, bacon, salami, hot dogs and some sausages. This was headline news; telling people to avoid all processed meats. The link between red and processed meat and cancer was further supported by a large scale study of over half a million people aged 50 to 71 years who were followed for 10 years (Sinha et al., 2009). They too found that red and processed meat intakes were associated with an increased risk of death from cancer (as well as cardiovascular disease).

The European Prospective Investigation into Cancer and Nutrition (EPIC) study is a Europe-wide prospective cohort study of the relationships between diet and cancer. With over half a million participants, it is the largest study of diet and disease to be undertaken. EPIC is coordinated by the International Agency for Research on Cancer (IARC), part of the World Health Organization (WHO). 521,457 healthy adults (mostly aged 35-70), were recruited from 23 centres in 10 European countries: Denmark, France, Germany, Greece, Italy, The Netherlands, Norway, Spain, Sweden and the UK. One UK centre (Oxford) recruited 27,000 vegetarians and vegans; this subgroup forms the largest study of this dietary group.

Strong evidence that vegetarian diets are associated with reduced cancer risk was provided by a recent large scale study from the Oxford Vegetarian Study and the EPIC-Oxford group. Prospective studies follow groups of people over time. Generally these people are alike in many but not all ways (for example, young women who smoke and young women who do not).

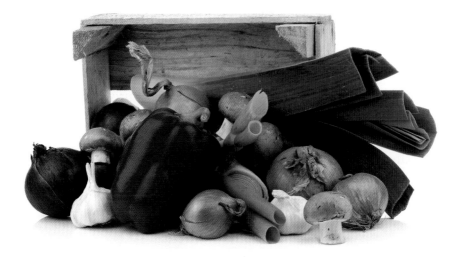

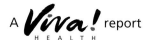
The prospective cohort study will then look for a link between their behaviour and a particular outcome (such as lung cancer). In this study, 61,566 British adults were separated into three diet groups: meat-eaters (32,403), fish-eaters (8,562) and vegetarians (20,601). After 12 years, 3,350 had been diagnosed with cancer (2,204 meat-eaters, 317 fish-eaters and 829 vegetarians). Total cancer incidence was significantly lower among both fish-eaters and vegetarians (18 and 12 per cent lower respectively) than among meat-eaters. Interestingly, there were vegans in this cohort, but there were too few to be informative (Key *et al.*, 2009). However, in a follow-on study, they determined a significant statistic for the vegan group; total cancer incidence was again lower in fish-eaters and vegetarians (12 and 11 per cent respectively) but was 19 per cent lower in vegans compared with meat-eaters (Key *et al.*, 2014).

Another large scale study (over 500,000 participants) from the EPIC group found that increasing the intake of fruit and vegetables by 200 grams per day lowered the risk of cancer (albeit by a few per cent). The authors cautioned against over interpreting these results when making dietary recommendations for cancer risk reduction because the magnitude of the effect was relatively small (Boffetta *et al.*, 2010). Both the vegetarian and non-vegetarian people in the EPIC-Oxford Study were shown to have overall lower cancer rates than the general population of the UK. It was noted that the meat intake of the meat-eaters group was lower than intakes reported in the National Diet and Nutrition Survey for the UK (Key *et al.*, 2009a). It seems likely that the meat-eaters in this health conscious study group are not typical of the wider meat-eating population. If you compared cancer rates between the average UK meat-eater with vegetarians and vegans, the difference between the two may be even greater.

The extent to which a vegetarian diet lowers the risk of cancer depends largely on what is in the diet. The diets of some Western vegetarians may have a similar macronutrient and micronutrient profile to that of a typical Western style diet. In other words, a vegetarian junk food diet! A wide variation exists in what Western vegetarians eat. The diet may include very large or very small amounts of: whole grain foods, raw foods, highly processed foods, sugary sweet foods, fatty foods and crucially may vary widely with respect to eggs, cheese, cream, butter and other dairy products. This may go some way to explain why there are discrepancies in the results of some studies looking at cancer and diet. This

(coupled to the 'health conscious' character of the meat-eaters in the EPIC group) may account for why a review of five prospective studies showed no large differences in cancer mortality between vegetarians and non-vegetarians (Key *et al.*, 1999). In another example from the EPIC group, they found that British vegetarians had a similar risk of colorectal cancer as non-vegetarians (Fraser *et al.*, 2009). Whereas other studies provide convincing evidence that plant-based diets are protective against colorectal cancer (WCRF/AICR, 2007). It is likely that using 'vegetarian' as a single dietary label in research is probably inadequate and this group needs to be divided into more descriptive subtypes to include vegans. However, taken together, the evidence suggests that vegetarian diets are a useful strategy for reducing cancer risk (Lanou and Svenson, 2010).

It has been suggested that animal protein increases the risk of cancer. In Professor T. Colin Campbell's extensive *China Study* (one of the largest studies in the world on the effects of diet on health) a startling observation was made. Based on previous work and his own studies, Campbell saw a direct link between dietary protein intake and cancer; the more protein in the diet, the higher the risk of certain cancers, such as liver cancer. But this was not all protein, just animal protein. Campbell decided to look at the relationships between animal protein intake and the incidence of cancer in different cultures.

Colorectal cancer is the fourth most common cancer in the world; it is the second most common in the US. Campbell noted that while North America, Europe, Australia and wealthier Asian countries (such as Japan and Singapore) had relatively high rates of colorectal cancer, Africa, Asia and most of Central and South America had much lower rates. For example, Campbell noted that the Czech Republic had a death rate of 34.19 per 100,000 males, while in Bangladesh the figure was just 0.63 per 100,000 males (Campbell and Campbell, 2005). Campbell is not alone in revealing the enormous differences in the incidences of certain cancers between countries. The International Agency for Research on Cancer (IARC) provides startling figures comparing the incidence of breast cancer and prostate cancer in England and Wales to that in rural China. In 1997, in England and Wales, the IARC reported the incidence rate of breast cancer in women was 68.8 per 100,000 compared to just 11.2 per 100,000 in rural China. Similarly the incidence of prostate cancer in men in England and Wales was 28.0 per 100,000 compared to just 0.5 per 100,000 in rural China (IARC, 1997).

Figure 4.0 A comparison of animal protein intake in the US, UK and rural China.

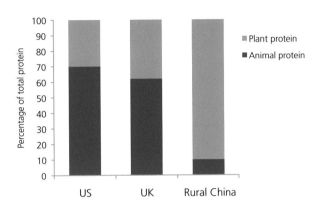

Source: Campbell and Campbell, 2005; Henderson *et al.*, 2003.

It is widely acknowledged that the incidence of certain cancers is much greater in some countries than others, what intrigued Campbell was the relationship between these cancers and dietary animal protein. Figure 4.0 shows the differences in animal protein intake between the US, the UK and rural China. In the US, over 15 per cent of total energy intake comes from protein of which 70 per cent is animal protein (Campbell and Campbell, 2005). In the UK, over 16 per cent of food energy comes from protein, and of this, 62 per cent comes from animal foods (Henderson *et al.*, 2003). While in rural China, the figures are quite different; nine to 10 per cent of total energy comes from protein and only 10 per cent of that is from animal protein (Campbell and Campbell, 2005).

It could be argued that the difference in cancer incidence between cultures reflects genetic differences between ethnic groups rather than environmental (dietary) effects. However, as stated above, migrant studies have shown that as people move from a low-cancer risk area to a high-cancer risk area, they assume an increased risk within two generations (WCRF/AICR, 1997). Therefore these vast differences in cancer rates must be largely attributable to environmental factors such as diet and lifestyle. Campbell concluded that animal-based foods are linked to an increased cancer risk whereas a whole grain plant-based diet including fibre and antioxidants is linked to lower rates of cancer (Campbell and Campbell, 2005). One possible mechanism for this may be the different composition of animal and plant proteins.

Plant proteins contain a different balance of amino acids than animal proteins. More specifically, plant

proteins contain less of the essential amino acids methionine and lysine than animal protein and more of the non-essential amino acids arginine, glycine, alanine and serine. It has been suggested that consuming mostly a plant-based diet has a knock-on effect of limiting the biological activity of certain chemical substances involved in cancer development and that a sufficient consumption of plant proteins has a protective role against cancer (Krajcovicova-Kudlackova, 2005). So a vegetarian diet is a healthier option, not just because it excludes meat and other animal foods but because of the range of beneficial, protective factors present. Vegetarian diets contain less saturated fats and more of the good fats (omega-3 and omega-6 unsaturated fatty acids), more complex carbohydrates, more fibre and more vitamins, minerals and antioxidants. These factors help to explain the reduced risk of cancer in vegetarians.

Increasing your fruit and vegetable consumption is considered the second most effective strategy to reduce the risk of cancer (after stopping smoking). Indeed, one of the most important messages of modern nutrition research is that a diet rich in fruits and vegetables protects not only against cancer, but against many other diseases too including heart disease and diabetes (Donaldson, 2004). In 2003 the UK Department of Health launched its 5-a-day campaign, encouraging people to eat more fruit and vegetables. The campaign is based on advice from the World Health Organization, which recommends eating a minimum of 400g of fruit and vegetables a day to lower the risk of serious health problems, such as heart disease, stroke, type 2 diabetes and obesity. In 2012 the National Diet and Nutrition Survey showed that despite the campaign, adults are still only eating four portions a day and children are eating just three or less.

Further to this, there is an increasing body of evidence linking the consumption of cow's milk to certain cancers. One of the reasons for this may be the increasing levels of hormones and other bioactive compounds present in the milk that result from intensive farming practices (taking milk from pregnant cows). In other words, in an effort to increase milk production, the dairy industry has intensified farming techniques to such a high level that between 75 per cent and 90 per cent of marketed milk and milk products are derived from pregnant cows (Danby, 2005). (See The undesirable components of milk and dairy products).

There are a number of other important factors that can contribute to the development of cancer, including

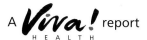

obesity (breast and endometrial cancer), alcohol (mouth, throat, liver and breast cancer), sunlight (skin cancer), radon (lung cancer) and physical activity can protect against some cancers (colorectal).

There are more than 200 different types of cancer, but just four of them (breast, lung, colorectal and prostate) account for over half (54 per cent) of all new cases (Cancer Research UK, 2012). The role of cow's milk and dairy products in breast, colorectal, ovarian and prostate cancer is discussed in more detail.

Breast cancer

Breast cancer is the most common cancer in the UK. When this report was first published in 2006, the lifetime risk of being diagnosed with breast cancer was one in nine for UK women. In 2014, the figure is one in eight. That means one in every eight women in the UK will develop breast cancer at some point in their lives. In the UK in 2010 more than 49,500 women and around 400 men were diagnosed with breast cancer, that's around 136 women per day and at least one man per day. Female breast cancer incidence rates in Britain have increased by almost 70 per cent since the mid-1970s. Just in the last ten years they have gone up by six per cent.

Figure 5.0 shows that while the incidence of breast cancer has risen sharply, mortality from breast cancer has fallen (albeit relatively modestly) over the same period thanks largely to improved diagnostic methods and more efficient treatment.

Much has been made of the link between genes and breast cancer. However, only five to ten per cent of all breast cancers are thought to be linked to an inherited breast cancer gene. The genes *BRCA1* and *BRCA2* have received the most attention since they were first discovered in 1994 and 1995 respectively. Between 45 and 90 out of every 100 women carrying BRCA genes will get breast cancer at some point in their lives. We now know of other genes that significantly increase a

woman's risk of breast cancer, they are called *TP53* and *PTEN*. Researchers have found other genes that can slightly increase a woman's risk of developing breast cancer, they include: *CASP8*, *FGFR2*, *TNRCP*, *MAP3K1*, *rs4973768*, *LSP1* and some rare genes that can also increase breast cancer risk slightly include: *CHEK2*, *ATM* (ataxia telangiectasia mutated), *BRIP1* and *PALB2* (MacMillan Cancer Support, 2011).

These discoveries linking genetics to cancer has given rise to a certain degree of genetic fatalism. However, as stated current estimates are that only around five to ten per cent of breast cancers are due to abnormal genes. This means that the vast majority of cancers (90-95 per cent) are not caused by abnormal genes. Secondly, it is important to remember that having an abnormal gene does not mean that a person will definitely develop breast cancer, but does mean they are considerably more at risk of developing the condition than someone who does not have one of the abnormal genes.

Lifestyle and environmental factors that can increase breast cancer risk include: age (the risk increases significantly as you get older), alcohol, obesity, early puberty, late menopause (women who have undergone the menopause have a lower risk of breast cancer than premenopausal women of the

Figure 5.0 Incidence of and mortality from breast cancer in England and Wales between 1971 and 2009.

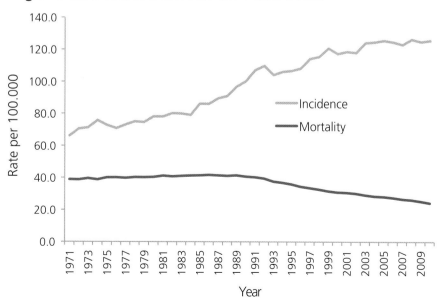

Source: National Statistics, 2010.

same age), late age at first childbirth, hormone replacement therapy (HRT) and the contraceptive pill. Factors that may decrease the risk include: younger age at first pregnancy (the younger the woman is when she begins childbearing, the lower her risk of breast cancer), breastfeeding, late puberty, early menopause and physical activity. The contribution of various environmental and lifestyle factors (excluding reproductive factors) to breast cancer risk has was calculated by a group from Harvard School of Public Health (Danaei et al., 2005). They conclude that 21 per cent of all breast cancer deaths worldwide are attributable to alcohol use, being overweight or obese and physical inactivity. This proportion is even higher (27 per cent) in high-income countries. That's nearly a third of all breast cancer cases being attributed to avoidable risk factors.

Breast cancer incidence rates vary greatly worldwide, with age standardised rates as high as 99.4 per 100,000 in North America. Eastern Europe, South America, Southern Africa and Western Asia have moderate incidence rates, but these are increasing. The lowest rates are found in most African countries but here breast cancer incidence rates are also increasing (WHO, 2013a). Migration studies show us that this variation is not due to genetic factors and that environmental and lifestyle factors must be involved. Because of this, an increasing amount of attention has focused on the links between diet and breast cancer, particularly the relationship between the consumption of cow's milk and dairy products and breast cancer.

Studying cancer incidence among particular groups of people can provide useful insights into the links between diet and disease. Researchers from the London School of Hygiene and Tropical Medicine recently reported breast cancer incidence is substantially lower, and survival rates higher, in South Asians living in the UK than other women (Farooq and Coleman, 2005). No data on diet was collected but the authors of this study suggested that differences in diet and lifestyle could explain the different rates observed. Earlier research published in the *British Journal of Cancer* also showed that South Asian women living in the UK are less likely to be diagnosed with breast cancer than other women, but found that the risk varied according to their specific ethnic subgroup. This research showed that Muslim women from India and Pakistan are almost twice as likely to develop breast cancer as Gujarati Hindu women. This study did examine the diet and found that the Gujarati Hindu women were more

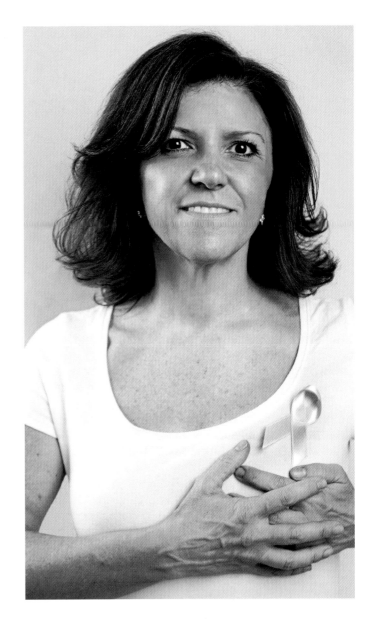

likely to be vegetarian and therefore had more fibre in their diet due to their higher intake of fruit and vegetables (McCormack et al., 2004). More recently, a prospective cohort study looked at the associations between plant foods, fibre and risk of breast cancer in 11,726 postmenopausal women in the Malmö Diet and Cancer cohort in Sweden among whom 342 incident cases of breast cancer were recorded. They found that a dietary pattern characterised by high fibre and low fat intakes was associated with a lower risk of postmenopausal breast cancer (Mattisson et al., 2009). There are several mechanisms by which fibre in the diet might influence breast cancer risk. One possible mechanism is through an effect on hormones: increasing the amount of fibre in the diet may reduce breast cancer risk by altering the levels of female hormones (oestrogens) circulating in the blood (Gerber, 1998).

A number of studies show that women with breast cancer tend to have higher levels of circulating oestrogens. A recent review of 13 studies concluded that circulating sex hormone concentrations in postmenopausal women are strongly associated with several established or suspected risk factors for breast cancer and may mediate the effects of these

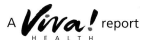

factors on breast cancer risk (Key *et al.*, 2011). In other words, some environmental or lifestyle factors (for example, obesity or alcohol consumption) may increase the levels of hormones circulating in the body and this may lead to breast cancer in some people.

A prospective study conducted on the island of Guernsey examined serum levels of the oestrogen hormone oestradiol in samples taken from 61 postmenopausal women who developed breast cancer an average of 7.8 years after blood collection. Compared to 179 age-matched controls, oestradiol levels were 29 per cent higher in women who later developed breast cancer (Thomas *et al.*, 1997). Another prospective study (this time from the US), compared oestrogen levels in 156 postmenopausal women who developed breast cancer, after blood collection, with two age-matched controls for each cancer patient. Results showed increased levels of the hormones oestradiol, oestrone, oestrone sulphate and dehydroepiandrosterone sulphate in women who subsequently developed breast cancer thus providing strong evidence for a causal relationship between postmenopausal oestrogen levels and the risk of breast cancer (Hankinson *et al.*, 1998). A review of studies carried out over a 10 year period in the Department of Clinical Chemistry at the University of Helsinki in Finland suggested that the Western diet (characterised by milk and meat products) increases levels of these types of hormones and concluded that the hormone pattern found in connection with a Western-type diet is prevailing in breast cancer patients (Adlercreutz, 1990).

Researchers at the Department of Preventive Medicine at the University of Southern California Medical School in Los Angeles published a review of 13 dietary fat intervention studies that were conducted to investigate the effect of fat intake on oestrogen levels. The results showed decreasing dietary fat intake (to between 10 and 25 per cent of the total energy intake) reduced serum oestradiol levels by between 2.7 and 10.3 per cent. It was concluded that dietary fat reduction can result in a lowering of serum oestradiol levels and that such a dietary modification may offer an approach to breast cancer prevention (Wu *et al.*, 1999). As stated, cow's milk and dairy products are a major source of dietary saturated fat.

These early reports are supported by more recent research that examined postmenopausal breast cancer risk in women consuming two different

dietary patterns in a large French cohort study. The 'alcohol/Western' diet included processed meat and meat products, ham, offal, French fries, appetisers, sandwiches, rice/pasta, potatoes, pulses, pizza/pies, canned fish, eggs, crustaceans, alcoholic beverages, cakes, mayonnaise, butter and cream and the 'healthy Mediterranean' diet was made up of a high intake of vegetables and fruits, fish and crustaceans, olives and sunflower oil. Results showed those eating the Western diet had a 20 per cent increased risk of breast cancer while those consuming the Mediterranean diet had a 15 per cent lower risk (Cottet *et al.*, 2009).

Identifying the type of diet that can increase or reduce the risk of cancer is just part of the puzzle. Identifying which components of that diet are responsible is another matter of considerable complexity. While some research has identified dietary factors that reduce the risk of breast cancer, such as fibre, other studies have attempted to identify dietary factors that increase the risk, such as dietary fat. Case-control studies use a group of people with a particular characteristic (for example older women with lung cancer). This particular group is selected and information collected (for example, history of smoking), then a control group is selected from a similar population (older women without lung cancer) to see if they smoked or not, then a conclusion is drawn (smoking does or does not increase risk of lung cancer). A combined analysis of 12 case-control studies designed to examine diet and breast cancer risk found a positive association between fat intake and this disease. The reviewers estimated that the percentage of breast cancers that might be prevented by dietary modification in the North American population was 24 per cent for postmenopausal women and 16 per cent for premenopausal women (Howe *et al.*, 1990). This is a significant number of cancers that could be prevented simply by changing the diet.

In a prospective cohort study involving over 90,000 premenopausal women, researchers from Harvard Medical School also found that animal fat intake was associated with an elevated risk of breast cancer. Red meat and high-fat dairy foods such as whole milk, cream, ice-cream, butter, cream cheese and cheese were the major contributors of animal fat in this cohort of relatively young women. Interestingly, this research did not find any clear association between vegetable fat and breast cancer risk; the increased risk was only associated with animal fat intake. It has been suggested that a high-fat diet increases the risk of breast cancer by elevating concentrations of oestrogen. However, the author of this study, Dr Eunyoung Cho, suggests that if this were true a diet high in animal fat and a diet high in vegetable fat should both lead to higher rates of cancer, and that was not the case in this study. Cho suspects that some other component such as the hormones in cow's milk might play a role in increasing the risk of breast cancer (Cho et al., 2003). A subsequent meta-analysis of all papers published up to July 2003 that examined the association of dietary fat with risk of breast cancer also found a positive association between higher intakes of fat and an increased risk of breast cancer (Boyd et al., 2003).

However, other studies of fat intake and the incidence of breast cancer have yielded conflicting results. The discrepancy in results may reflect the difficulties of accurately recording fat intake. Dr Sheila Bingham of the Dunn Human Nutrition Unit in Cambridge developed a data-collection method to overcome these problems. Bingham used food frequency questionnaire methods with a detailed seven-day food diary in over 13,000 women between 1993 and 1997. The study concluded that those who ate the most animal saturated fat (found mainly in whole milk, butter, meat, cakes and biscuits) were almost twice as likely to develop breast cancer as those who ate the least. It was also concluded that previous studies may have failed to establish this link because of imprecise methods (Bingham et al., 2003). That said, a recent study using data from four prospective cohort studies in the United Kingdom (EPIC-Norfolk , EPIC-Oxford, the UKWCS and Whitehall II study) found no association between dietary fat and breast cancer (Key et al., 2011a). These researchers were aware of the methodology problems identified by Bingham and could not identify any reason why their results were different from those of Bingham's group. More research is needed to clarify the role of total fat and saturated fat in breast cancer.

Some research groups are more interested in the endogenous hormonal content of milk (hormones produced by the cow and excreted in the milk), which has not been widely discussed. The milk produced now is very different from that produced 100 years ago; modern dairy cows are impregnated while still producing milk (Webster, 2005). **Two-thirds of milk in the UK is taken from pregnant cows with the remainder coming from cows that have recently given birth**. This means that the hormone (oestrogen, progesterone and androgen

precursor) content of milk varies widely. It is the high levels of hormones in milk that have been linked to the development of hormone-dependent cancers such as ovarian and breast cancer.

In a review of the relationship between breast cancer incidence and food intake among the populations of 40 different countries, a positive correlation was seen between the consumption of meat, milk and cheese and the incidence of breast (and ovarian) cancer. Meat was most closely correlated with breast cancer incidence, followed by cow's milk and cheese. By contrast, cereals and pulses were negatively correlated with the incidence of breast cancer. This review concluded that the increased consumption of animal foods may have adverse effects on the development of hormone-dependent cancers. Among dietary risk factors of particular concern were milk and dairy products, because so much of the milk we drink today is taken from pregnant cows, in which oestrogen and progesterone levels are markedly elevated (Ganmaa and Sato, 2005). Commercial milk products have been shown to contain considerable levels of oestrogen metabolites (Farlow et al., 2009). This raises concerns that the high levels of oestrogen metabolites and other bioactive molecules in milk may influence cancer risk.

In a review of the evidence linking dairy consumption to breast cancer risk, researchers from Princeton University in New Jersey concluded that milk may promote breast cancer by the action of the growth factor IGF-1, which has been shown to stimulate the growth of human breast cancer cells in the laboratory (Outwater et al., 1997). In another review, examining the role of IGF-1 in cancer development, Yu and Rohan state that IGFs play a critical role in regulating cell growth and death. This function has led to speculation about their involvement in cancer development. Laboratory experiments demonstrate the ability of IGFs to stimulate growth of a wide range of cancer cells and to suppress cell death or apoptosis (Yu and Rohan, 2000). The concern here is that if IGF-1 can cause human cancer cells to grow in a Petri dish in the laboratory, they might have a cancer-inducing effect when consumed in the diet. Furthermore, cow's milk is known to increase IGF-1 levels in the blood by driving up IGF-1 production by the liver.

IGF-1 is present in all milk and is not destroyed during pasteurisation. Dr J.L. Outwater of the Physicians Committee For Responsible Medicine (PCRM) in Washington, DC, warns that IGF-1 may be

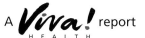

absorbed across the gut and cautions that regular milk ingestion after weaning may produce enough IGF-1 in mammary tissue to encourage cell division thus increasing the risk of cancer (Outwater *et al.*, 1997). However, other scientists contest this view and say that IGF-1 could not cross the gut wall at sufficient levels to alter systemic levels already circulating but do say that there are many small peptides and amino acids that are present in milk that potently stimulate hepatic IGF-1 expression and pituitary growth hormone release (Holly, 2013). In either scenario, the net effect is the same; cow's milk consumption raises IGF-1 levels in humans and higher IGF-1 levels are linked to cancers of the colon, prostate and breast.

In her book *Your Life in Your Hands*, Professor Jane Plant CBE, the chief scientist of the British Geological Survey, describes a very personal and moving story of how she overcame breast cancer by excluding all dairy products from her diet (Plant, 2007). Plant was diagnosed with breast cancer in 1987. She had five recurrences of the disease and by 1993 the cancer had spread to her lymphatic system. She could feel the lump on her neck, and was told that she had just three months to live, six if she was lucky. However, Plant was determined to use her scientific training to find a solution to this 'problem'. She began

researching breast cancer in other cultures and found a much lower incidence in China. The data showed that in rural China breast cancer affects just one in 10,000 women compared to one in 10 British women (now one in eight). However, Plant observed that among wealthy Chinese women with a more Western lifestyle (for example in Malaysia and Singapore), the rate of breast cancer is similar to that in the West. Furthermore, epidemiological evidence shows that when Chinese women move to the West, within one or two generations their rates of breast cancer incidence and mortality increase to match those of their host country. This suggested that diet and lifestyle (rather than genetics) must be a major determinant of cancer risk.

Plant decided to investigate the role of diet in breast cancer risk. She examined the results of the China-Cornell-Oxford project on nutrition, environment and health (Campbell and Junshi, 1994). This project was based on national surveys conducted between 1983 and 1984 in China. The project was a collaboration between T. Colin Campbell at Cornell University in the US, Chen Junshi from the Chinese Academy of Preventative Medicine, in Beijing, China, Li Junyao at the Chinese Academy of Medical Sciences, Beijing, and Richard Peto from Oxford University in the UK. The project revealed some surprising insights into

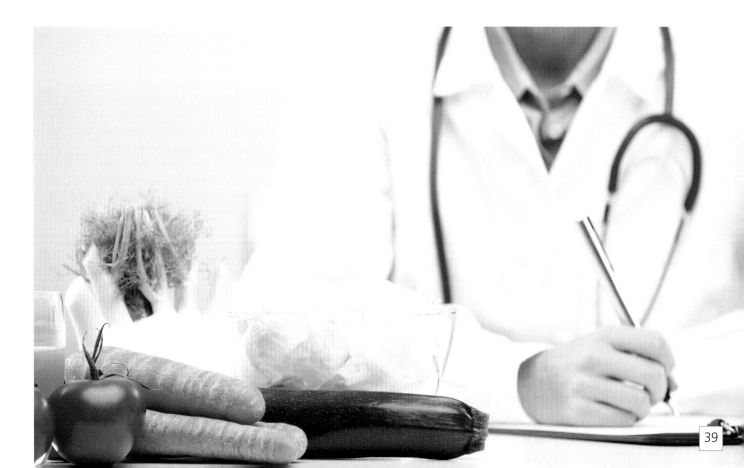

diet and health. For example, it showed that people in China tend to consume more calories per day that people in the US, but only 14 per cent of these calories come from fat compared to a massive 36 per cent in the West. This coupled to the fact that Chinese people tend to be more physically active than people in the West, is why obesity affects far more people in the West than in China. However, Plant's diet had not been particularly high in fat; indeed she describes it as very low in fat and high in fibre. Then Plant had a revelation: the Chinese don't eat dairy produce. Plant had been eating yogurt and skimmed organic milk up until this time, but within days of ceasing all dairy, the lump on her neck began to shrink. The tumour decreased and eventually disappeared, leading her to the conviction that there is a causal link between the consumption of dairy products and breast cancer. Although Plant received chemotherapy during this time, it did not appear to be working and so convinced was her cancer

specialist that it was the change in diet that saved her life, he now refers to cancer mortality maps in his lectures and recommends a dairy-free diet to his breast cancer patients.

Plant eventually defeated cancer by eliminating dairy products from her diet, replacing them with healthy alternatives and making some lifestyle changes. At the time of writing (2007) Plant had been cancer-free for 14 years and now advises that if you do only one thing to cut your risk of breast cancer, make the change from dairy to soya (Plant, 2007).

A meta-analysis of the effects of soya on breast cancer found a mildly protective rather than deleterious effect in premenopausal women (Trock *et al.*, 2006) and more recently a paper from the Shanghai Breast Cancer study also indicated somewhat better outcomes related to soya consumption in woman with established breast cancer Shu *et al.*, 2009). Providing breast cancer patients with sound dietary advice could greatly increase survival rates. Taken together, these observations show that a dairy-free plant-based diet can reduce many of the risk factors associated with breast cancer and may help those who have been diagnosed with the disease.

Colorectal (bowel) cancer

Colorectal cancer is the second most common cancer in England and the third most common cause of cancer death (after lung and prostate cancer in men, and lung and breast cancer in women). Between 1971 and 2009 the incidence of colorectal cancer increased by 33 per cent for men and 14 per cent for women. In 2009 there were 18,538 new cases for men and 15,066 for women. While the incidence of colorectal cancer has increased, mortality rates have halved for women between 1971 and 2010 and have decreased by 38 per cent for men during this time. In 2010, there were 15,708 deaths from bowel cancer in the UK: 8,574 (55 per cent) in men and 7,134 (45 per cent) in women (Office for National Statistics, 2012). Colorectal cancer occurs when the process of cell renewal in the bowel goes wrong. Abnormal cells can form polyps (small growths) which may develop into cancer. Risk factors for colorectal cancer include obesity, alcohol, smoking and poor diet.

A large body of evidence suggests a diet high in red and processed meat (such as smoked meat, ham,

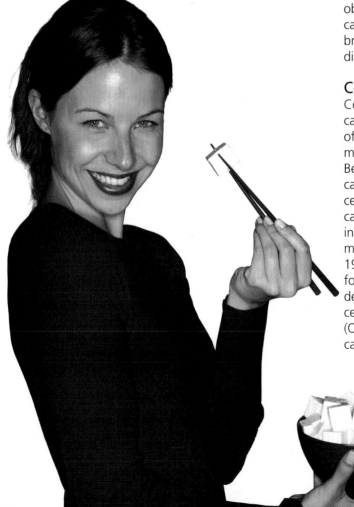

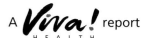

bacon, sausages, pâté and tinned meat) can increase the risk of colorectal cancer. In 2005, a large prospective study from the EPIC group investigated the role of diet in colorectal cancer. They followed 478,040 men and women from 10 European countries between 1992 and 1998. Information on diet and lifestyle was collected and after nearly five years, 1,329 cases of colorectal cancer were recorded. Results showed that colorectal cancer risk is linked to a high consumption of red and processed meat (Norat *et al*., 2005). Several mechanisms by which red and processed meat may cause colorectal cancer have been suggested. The type of iron (haem iron) found in meat, but not plant foods, may cause changes in cells that lead to cancer (Tapel *et al*., 2007). Other compounds found in red and processed meats called N-nitroso compounds, heterocyclic amines and polycyclic aromatic hydrocarbons may be responsible for the link with cancer (Lewin *et al*., 2006; Cross *et al*., 2007; Genkinger and Koushik, 2007).

In November 2007, The World Cancer Research Fund launched the report *Food, Nutrition, Physical Activity, and the Prevention of Cancer: a Global Perspective*. It was the most comprehensive report to date ever published on the link between cancer and lifestyle (WCRF/AICR, 2007). Their recommendation to eat less red meat (such as beef, pork and lamb) and avoid processed meat became headline news on a global scale. In more detail, they said: To reduce your cancer risk, eat no more than 500 grams (cooked weight) per week of red meat, like beef, pork and lamb, and avoid processed meats such as ham, bacon, salami, hot dogs and some sausages. The report warned that eating 150 grams of processed meat a day (the equivalent of two sausages and three rashers of bacon) increases bowel cancer risk by 63 per cent and that 50 grams a day (one sausage) increases the risk by about 20 per cent. The evidence that processed meat is a cause of bowel cancer is so strong that the WCRF recommends that people should avoid eating it altogether. However, less than a third of people in Britain are aware that eating processed meat such as bacon and ham increases risk of cancer (WCRF, 2009). 10 per cent of bowel cancers cases in the UK could be prevented through reducing the amount of processed meat we eat. The Department of Health advises people who eat more than 90 grams (cooked weight) of red and processed meat per day to cut down on their intake (NHS Choices, 2012e).

While red and processed meat is linked to an increased risk of colorectal cancer, there is good evidence that a diet high in fibre and low in saturated fat can help reduce the risk (NHS Choices, 2012e). Several mechanisms by which fibre may offer a protective effect have been suggested: the formation of short-chain fatty acids from fermentation by colonic bacteria; the reduction of secondary bile acid production; the reduction in intestinal transit time and increase of faecal bulk; and a reduction in insulin resistance (Murphy *et al*., 2012).

The protective role of a whole grain plant-based diet containing plenty of fruit and vegetables (and therefore fibre) is well-documented. Two large-scale studies (both published in the *Lancet*) examined the relationship between diet and colorectal cancer; both confirmed that as dietary fibre intake increases, the risk of colorectal cancer decreases. In the first of these two studies, a research team from the National Cancer Institute in the US compared fibre intake of 3,591 people with at least one bowel adenoma or polyp (a benign growth that may or may not transform to cancer), with that of 33,971 people without polyps. They found that the participants in the top 20 per cent for dietary fibre intake had 27 per cent lower risk of adenoma than people in the lowest 20 per cent (representing a difference in fibre intake of 24 grams per day). It was concluded that dietary fibre, particularly from grains, cereals and fruits, was associated with a decreased risk of colorectal adenoma (Peters *et al*., 2003). In the second study, (the largest prospective study published at that time on fibre in colorectal cancer prevention) researchers from the EPIC group prospectively examined the association between dietary fibre intake and incidence of colorectal cancer in 519,978 individuals aged between 25 and 70 years-old, recruited from 10 different European countries. Participants completed a dietary questionnaire between 1992 and 1998 and were followed up for cancer incidence on average 4.5 years later. From this group, 1,065 cases of colorectal cancer were reported. Again, people with the highest fibre intake (35 grams per day) had a 40 per cent lower risk of colorectal cancer compared to those with the lowest intake (15 grams per day). They concluded that in populations with low average intake of dietary fibre, an approximate doubling of total fibre intake from foods could reduce the risk of colorectal cancer by 40 per cent (Bingham *et al*., 2003a). These studies provide convincing evidence that increasing the amount of whole grains and fruit and vegetables in the diet reduces the risk of colorectal cancer. A further EPIC report, in which an even larger number of cases (1,721 cases) were included, confirmed the original results showing an even stronger protective association between fibre intake in food and risk of colorectal cancer (Bingham *et al.*, 2005). In the most recent EPIC study, 4,517 colorectal cancer cases were documented amongst the 477,312 participants (Murphy *et al.*, 2012). After 11 years of follow-up, this analysis of EPIC data also confirmed the protective role of dietary fibre in colorectal cancer.

Not all studies report a positive effect of fibre; some have found that fibre has little or no effect on colorectal cancer risk (Pietinen *et al.*, 1999; Fuchs, *et al.*, 1999; Terry *et al.*, 2001). It should be noted that these studies only looked at populations from single countries and may have looked at ranges of fibre that were too low. For example, Americans eat very little fibre on average. So a large study that focused on Americans would not be able to see the benefits of the high levels of fibre that, for example, an Italian person would eat (Cancer Research UK, 2009). Taken together, the WCRF and EPIC research (which looks at multiple countries) and numerous other studies (Jacobs *et al.*, 1998; Peters *et al.*, 2003; Nomura *et al.*, 2007; Wakai *et al.*, 2007) confirm the protective role of dietary fibre intake in colorectal cancer. These results strengthen the evidence for the recommendation of increasing the consumption of fibre rich foods for colorectal cancer prevention.

Studies looking at the links between dairy foods and colorectal cancer have produced mixed results. Some prospective studies have reported a lower colorectal cancer risk associated with dairy products and calcium. In 2004, a pooled analysis of 10 cohort studies from North America and Europe concluded that the consumption of dairy milk (but not other dairy foods) and calcium were related to a lower risk of colorectal cancer (Cho *et al.*, 2004). The inverse association between calcium intake and colorectal cancer was only statistically significant among those with the highest vitamin D intake. This may be either because vitamin D enhances calcium absorption, or because vitamin D itself may decrease colorectal cancer risk (Garland, 1999). More recently, an updated meta-analysis from the WCRF Continuous Update Project also found that milk and total dairy products (but not cheese or other dairy products), are associated with a reduction in colorectal cancer risk (Aune *et al.*, 2012).

The principal anti-carcinogenic component in cow's milk and dairy products is believed to be calcium (Murphy *et al.*, 2013). One study looking at dairy foods and calcium intakes in relation to cancer in the National Institutes of Health (NIH)-AARP (formerly known as the American Association of Retired Persons) Diet and Health Study found that during an average of seven years of follow-up, dairy food and calcium intakes were inversely associated with cancers of the digestive system. A decreased risk was particularly pronounced in colorectal cancer. Interestingly in this study, supplemental calcium intake was also inversely associated with colorectal cancer risk. They concluded that calcium intake is associated with a lower risk of total cancer and cancers of the digestive system, especially colorectal cancer (Park *et al.*, 2009). A meta-analysis of 60 epidemiological studies including 26,335 colorectal cases also found that the risk reduction associated with calcium was similar for dietary and supplemental sources (Huncharek *et al.*, 2009). So in these studies, it would appear to be the calcium rather than some unidentified component of dairy that lowered the risk.

However, the EPIC group found that their inverse associations were limited to dairy sources of calcium. They investigated intakes of milk (whole-fat, semi-skimmed and skimmed), yoghurt, cheese and dietary calcium with colorectal cancer risk amongst 477,122 men and women. During 11 years of follow-up, 4,513 incident cases of colorectal cancer occurred. Results showed that higher intakes of all dairy products and dietary calcium (from dairy sources only) were associated with a modest (seven per cent) reduction in colorectal cancer risk (Murphy *et al.*, 2013). They suggest that a possible explanation for the lack of a protective effect of non-dairy calcium could be that plant sources of calcium (the main contributors to non-dairy calcium intake amongst EPIC participants) contain oxalate and phytate (phytic acid) which inhibit calcium absorption. Furthermore, it should be noted that dietary calcium has been consistently associated with an increased risk of prostate cancer risk. Within EPIC, a 300 mg per day intake of dietary calcium was previously associated with a nine per cent increased risk of prostate cancer (Allen *et al.*, 2008) and the WCRF/AICR 2007 report judged it a probable cause of the disease (WCRF/AICR, 2007). So it would seem clear that recommending dairy to men to lower their risk of colorectal cancer would not be a sensible option. Indeed, obtaining a good supply of calcium from non-oxalate vegetables and other plant-based foods (see below) is the healthier option for all people.

It has been suggested that the high-fat content of some dairy products may negate their protective effect against certain cancers. However the EPIC

Calcium-rich foods

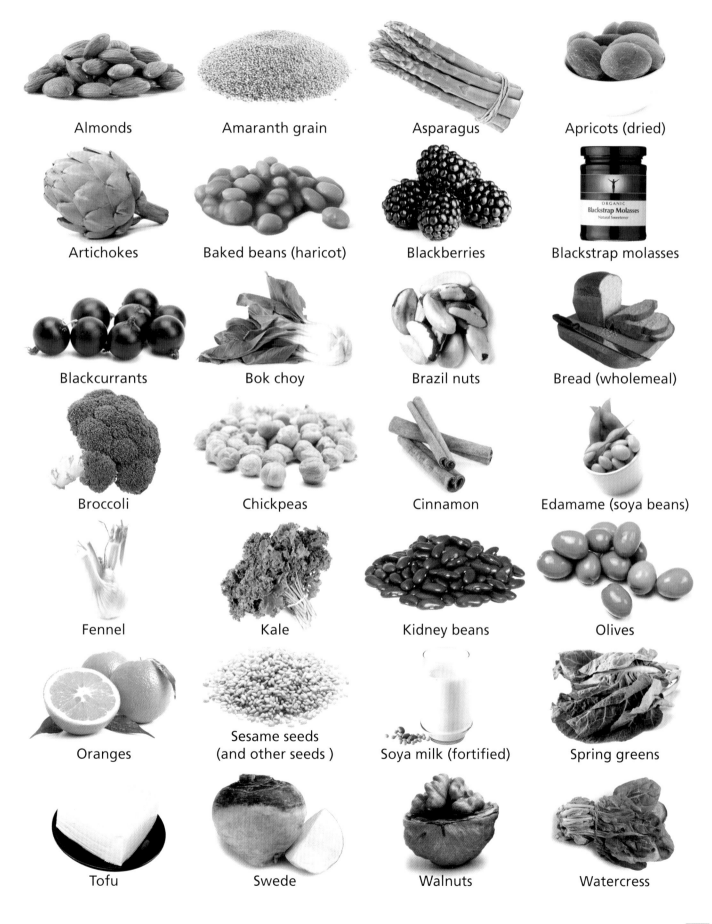

Almonds	Amaranth grain	Asparagus	Apricots (dried)
Artichokes	Baked beans (haricot)	Blackberries	Blackstrap molasses
Blackcurrants	Bok choy	Brazil nuts	Bread (wholemeal)
Broccoli	Chickpeas	Cinnamon	Edamame (soya beans)
Fennel	Kale	Kidney beans	Olives
Oranges	Sesame seeds (and other seeds)	Soya milk (fortified)	Spring greens
Tofu	Swede	Walnuts	Watercress

study found no difference in how high or low-fat dairy products affected colorectal cancer risk (Murphy *et al*, 2013). Other constituents of dairy products may contribute to the protective role observed. For example lactoferrin, vitamin D in fortified dairy products and certain fatty acids, such as butyric acid, have been linked with having possible beneficial roles against colorectal cancer (Murphy *et al.*, 2013). Also it should be noted that in the EPIC cohort the lowest dairy consumers had the highest proportion of smokers and the highest dairy consumers were more physically active, had lower BMIs, had lower intakes of alcohol, higher intakes of fibre and had achieved a higher level of education. Because we have been led to believe that milk is a health food, it may be that people who use dairy may be doing other 'healthy' activities which could be masking the negative effects of their dairy consumption, even making it look positively healthy. More work is required to tease out these complex relationships.

As with breast cancer, there are growing concerns that the consumption of cow's milk raises levels of IGF-1 in the blood (either directly or indirectly) and higher IGF-1 levels are a risk factor for colorectal cancer. In fact, circulating IGF-1 levels are not just related to future colorectal cancer risk but may also predict cancer progression (Renehan *et al.*, 2001). In a study of 204 healthy men and women aged 55 to 85 years, three servings of non-fat milk per day over 12 weeks increased blood serum levels of IGF-1 by 10 per cent (Heaney, 1999). Because elevated levels of IGF-1 are associated with increased risk of colorectal cancer (Ma *et al.*, 1999; Giovannucci *et al.*, 2000; Kaaks *et al.*, 2000), an increase in IGF-1 attributable to the consumption of milk could potentially counter any protective effect conferred by dietary calcium (and vitamin D in US fortified milk).

Taken together, the research suggests that plant foods provide a safer and healthier source of calcium than dairy products. Plant-based sources of calcium, including non-oxalate dark green leafy vegetables, dried fruits, nuts, seeds and pulses as well as fortified foods such as calcium-set tofu (soya bean curd) and calcium-enriched soya milk, provide a safer source of calcium. Vitamin D can be either obtained from the diet or synthesised in the skin following exposure to sunlight.

To lower your risk of colorectal cancer it is important to eat a healthy plant-based diet rich in fibre and low in fat, take regular physical exercise, maintain a healthy weight and avoid excessive alcohol consumption and avoid smoking.

Ovarian cancer

The ovaries are two almond shaped organs located on either side of the uterus. They produce eggs and the reproductive hormones (oestrogen and progesterone). Ovarian cancer affects more than 6,500 women in the UK each year. It is the fifth most common cancer among women after breast cancer, bowel cancer, lung cancer and cancer of the uterus (NHS Choices, 2012f).

Several possible risk factors for ovarian cancer have been identified. Most ovarian cancers are due to gene changes that develop during a woman's life but about one in 10 ovarian cancers are caused by an inherited faulty gene. Faulty inherited genes that increase the risk of ovarian cancer include *BRCA1* and *BRCA2*; these genes also increase the risk of breast cancer (Cancer Research UK, 2012a). As with most cancers, the risk of developing ovarian cancer increases as you get older. Most cases are in women who have had their menopause.

Apart from getting older, the risk of ovarian cancer may be increased by a range of actors including:

- A family history of cancer
- Having breast cancer
- Being infertile or having fertility treatment
- Using a coil (intra uterine device – IUD)
- Using hormone replacement therapy (HRT)
- Being overweight or tall
- Having endometriosis
- Using talcum powder
- Smoking
- Diet factors

Source: Cancer Research UK, 2012a.

It has been suggested that the milk sugar lactose is a risk factor for ovarian cancer. A positive relationship between ovarian cancer and dairy products was first reported in the Lancet in 1989 when it was suggested that lactose consumption may be a dietary risk factor for ovarian cancer (Cramer *et al.*, 1989). In 2004, data collected from the Harvard Nurses' Health Study was used to assess the lactose, milk and milk product consumption in relation to ovarian cancer risk in over 80,000 women. Over 16 years of follow-up, 301 cases of one particular type of ovarian cancer were confirmed in this study group. Results showed that women who consumed the most lactose had twice the risk of this type of ovarian cancer than women who drank the least lactose. It was suggested that galactose (a

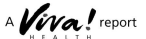

component of lactose) may damage ovarian cells making them more susceptible to cancer (Fairfield *et al.*, 2004).

In the same year, Susanna Larsson and colleagues of the Karolinska Institute in Stockholm, Sweden, published a study in the *American Journal of Clinical Nutrition* that examined the association between intakes of dairy products and lactose and the risk of ovarian cancer. In this study of 61,084 women aged 38 to 76 years, the diet was assessed over three years and after 13.5 years 266 participants had been diagnosed with ovarian cancer. Results showed that women consuming four or more servings of dairy a day had double the risk of ovarian cancer compared to low or non-dairy consumers. Milk was the dairy product with the strongest positive association with ovarian cancer. The authors of this study observed a positive association between lactose intake and ovarian cancer risk and concluded that high intakes of lactose and dairy products, particularly milk, are associated with an increased risk of ovarian cancer (Larsson *et al.*, 2004).

Larsson subsequently compared two groups of studies: three prospective cohort studies and 18 case-control studies. The results of the three prospective cohort studies showed a strong link between the intake of total dairy foods, low-fat milk and lactose and the risk of ovarian cancer. In contrast, the data from the 18 case-control studies produced mixed results and (except for whole milk, which was consistently linked to an increased risk of ovarian cancer) these studies did not provide evidence of a positive association between dairy food and lactose intake with ovarian cancer (Larsson *et al.*, 2006). The differences between the findings of the cohort and case-control studies might be explained by a number of factors including selection bias (choosing individuals that are not representative of the norm) or changes in the diet following cancer diagnosis. Alternatively, the differences between the findings may be due to the time interval between diet assessment and cancer diagnosis. Cohort studies frequently record dietary practices many years before illness occurs, which may make the data more likely to be accurate compared to data collected in case-control studies which tends to be collected at the time of diagnosis.

In another study examining the link between diet and ovarian cancer, ovarian cancer incidence between 1993 and 1997 in different geographical locations was coupled to food consumption data from FAOSTAT Database Collections. The food items used for this study were animal fats, meat (beef,

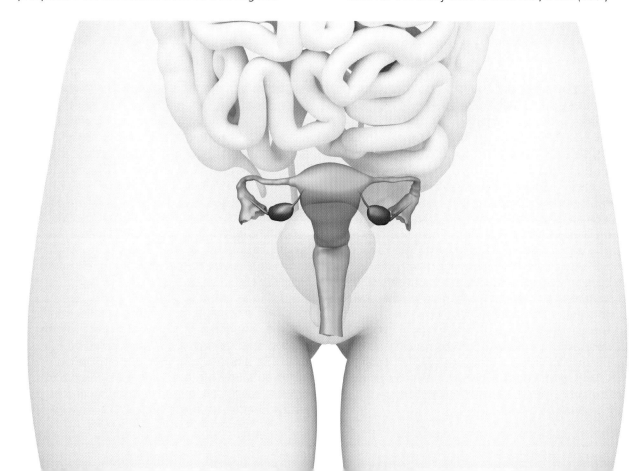

pork, poultry, mutton and goat meat), eggs, butter, milk, cereals, pulses, beans, soya beans, peas, fruits, vegetables, coffee, tea and alcoholic beverages. Results showed that Iceland had the highest rates of ovarian cancer affecting 16.2 women per 100,000, followed by 15.2 in Sweden and 13.7 in the UK. The lowest rate per 100,000 was 1.6 for Korea, followed by 2.1 in Mali and 4.0 in both China and Brazil. Again, results showed a strong link between dairy foods and cancer: milk was most closely correlated with the incidence of ovarian cancer, followed by animal fats and cheese. Conversely, pulses were negatively correlated with the incidence of this cancer (Ganmaa and Sato, 2005). This provides yet more evidence that animal-based foods tend to increase the risk of disease while whole grain plant-based diets reduce the risk.

While several other studies have shown that dairy intake increases ovarian cancer risk, other studies have found no evidence of an association. A number of epidemiological studies have also examined the influence of specific nutrients from dairy products, including lactose, calcium and fat in the development of ovarian cancer. However, results from these studies are also mixed. In an effort to resolve this uncertainty, scientists from The Danish Cancer Society Research Center investigated the association between intake of specific dairy products and related nutrients (lactose and calcium) and ovarian cancer risk in a large population-based case-control study among Danish women. They found that the intake of dairy products (particularly milk, soured milk products and yoghurt), was associated with an increased overall ovarian cancer risk. A similar association was found between lactose intake and overall ovarian cancer risk (Faber *et al.*, 2012).

In conclusion, the consumption of animal-based foods is associated with an increased risk of certain hormone-dependent cancers. Milk and dairy products are of particular concern: as already stated, most milk drunk today is produced from pregnant cows, in which oestrogen and progesterone levels are markedly elevated (Ganmaa and Sato, 2005). While there are several candidate components of milk that may increase the risk of ovarian and other hormone-dependent cancers, the precise mechanisms underlying their action remain unclear. However, as milk and dairy products have been identified as a risk factor for ovarian cancer, it stands to reason that this particular risk can be reduced by switching to a plant-based diet that excludes all dairy products.

Prostate cancer

Prostate cancer is the most common cancer in men in the UK, with over 40,000 new cases diagnosed every year (NHS Choices, 2012g). It is the second most common cause of cancer death in UK men, after lung cancer (Cancer Research UK, 2012b). In the UK, about one in nine men will get prostate cancer at some point in their lives. This lifetime risk includes men who get prostate cancer at any age and more than half of all cases are diagnosed in men over 70, prostate cancer is quite rare in men under 50 (Cancer Research UK, 2012c).

Prostate cancer develops from cells within the prostate gland which is the size of a walnut and lies directly under the bladder. The prostate produces a protein called prostate-specific antigen (PSA) which turns semen into liquid form. The majority of prostate cancers are slow growing and it may be some time before any symptoms are noticed, which can make this disease less treatable. Symptoms include: needing to urinate often, especially at night; difficulty starting to urinate; straining to urinate or taking a long time to finish and pain when urinating or during sex. Other less common symptoms include: pain in the lower back and blood in the urine.

Cancer is not usually inherited, but some types (breast, ovarian and prostate cancer) can be influenced by genes and can run in families. Having a close male relative (such as a brother, father or uncle) who has had prostate cancer can be linked to an increased risk. Men who have relatives with breast cancer (especially under the age of 60) may also have a higher risk of prostate cancer. This increased risk may be caused by inherited faulty genes *BRCA1* and *BRCA2*. Men who carry a faulty *BRCA1* gene may have a slightly higher risk (one per cent) of male breast cancer. Some studies suggest there may be a slight increase in the risk of prostate cancer. Men who carry a faulty *BRCA2* gene have a seven per cent higher chance of getting breast cancer and a 20-25 per cent higher lifetime risk of developing prostate cancer. Most of these prostate cancers occur over the age of 45 (Oxford University Hospitals NHS Trust, 2011).

There are many different factors that influence the development of prostate cancer Experts think that just five to 15 per cent of prostate cancers are linked to inherited genes (Macmillan Cancer Support, 2013a). That means that 85 per cent or more of prostate cancers are caused by environmental and/or lifestyle factors. Research suggests there may be a

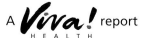

link between obesity and prostate cancer and that men who regularly exercise have a lower risk of developing the disease. Some evidence suggests that diet can affect your risk of developing prostate cancer. Current thinking suggests that a diet high in animal fats may increase your risk of developing prostate cancer. In particular, red meat (such as beef, lamb and pork), eggs and dairy produce (including butter, whole milk, cheese and cream) contain a lot of saturated fat (Macmillan Cancer Support, 2013a). As we see with other hormone-dependent cancers (for example, breast cancer), the highest incidence rates of prostate cancer occur in the developed world and the lowest rates are seen in Africa and Asia. However, African-American men are more affected than white American men. This suggests that prostate cancer risk is influenced by dietary and lifestyle factors.

Figure 6.0 shows how the incidence of prostate cancer varies widely around the world. Incidence rates are highest in Australia, New Zealand and Western Europe (104 and 93 per 100,000 in 2008 respectively), where prostate cancer screening and PSA testing is common. The lowest rates are seen in South-Central Asia; four per 100,000 (Cancer Research UK, 2012d).

Research shows that prostate cancer rates are lower in countries with low consumption rates of typical Western foods such as meat and dairy. However, advice from the NHS on the links between diet and prostate cancer is fairly sparse. They say that there is evidence that a diet high in calcium is linked to an increased risk of developing prostate cancer and that some research has shown prostate cancer rates appear lower in men who eat foods containing certain nutrients including lycopene, found in tomatoes and other red fruit, and selenium, found in Brazil nuts (NHS Choices, 2012h).

It is now well-documented that diets high in calcium and dairy protein can increase the risk of prostate cancer (Cancer Research UK, 2012c). One of the earliest reports linking dairy consumption to prostate cancer was published in the 1980s when a study of over 27,000 Californian Seventh-Day Adventists who had completed dietary questionnaires 20 years earlier concluded that milk consumption was positively associated with prostate cancer mortality (Snowdon, 1988). Since then many more reports have confirmed an increased risk from the consumption of dairy foods.

One possible mechanism for the action of milk in increasing prostate cancer risk may involve the calcium in milk. Researchers from Harvard Medical School have shown that high consumption of calcium is linked to advanced prostate cancer (Giovannucci et al., 1998). It has been suggested that calcium increases prostate cancer risk by suppressing circulating vitamin D (Giovannucci, 1998). In a study of 3,612 men observed between 1982 and 1992, 131 prostate cancer cases were identified and dietary intake analysed (Tseng et al., 2005). Results confirmed that dietary calcium was associated with an increased risk whereas vitamin D was not associated. The researchers concluded that dairy consumption may increase prostate cancer risk through a calcium-related pathway.

Figure 6.0 Incidence and mortality rates for prostate cancer in selected countries in 2008.

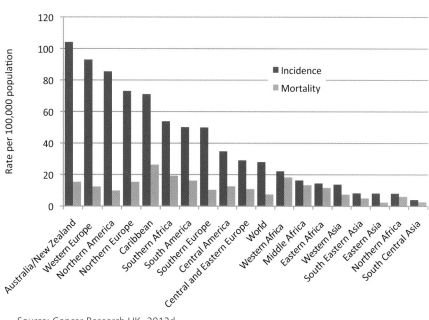

Source: Cancer Research UK, 2012d.

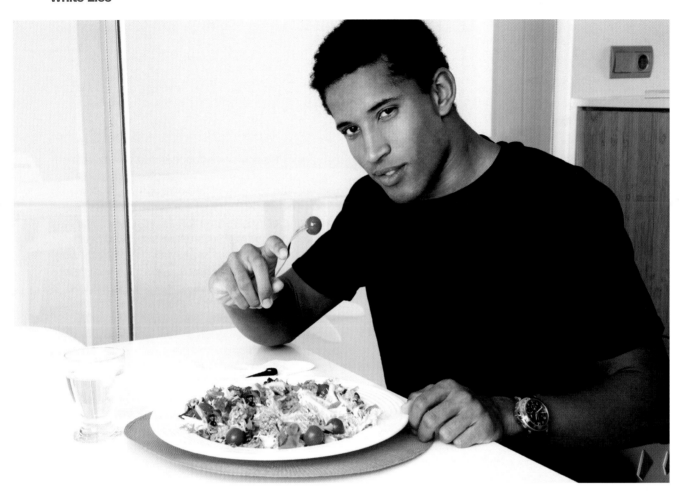

More recently an EPIC study found that a 35g per day increase in consumption of dairy protein was associated with a 32 per cent increase in the risk of prostate cancer. They also found that calcium from dairy products was positively associated with risk, but not calcium from other foods. These results support the hypothesis that a high intake of protein or calcium from dairy products may increase the risk for prostate cancer (Allen *et al.*, 2008). Given that calcium and low-fat milk are vigorously promoted to reduce risk of osteoporosis (and colon cancer), the mechanisms by which dairy and calcium might increase prostate cancer risk should be clarified and confirmed (Tseng *et al.*, 2005).

Another study considered the oestrogen content of milk as a causal factor, having noted that the typical Western diet (characterised by milk and meat products) contains higher levels of oestrogen than the foods eaten by Asian men who suffer much less from prostate cancer. This study measured the hormone contents of two kinds of commercial milks (from Holstein and Jersey cows) and found that levels were markedly higher than they were 20 years ago. This was attributed to modern dairy farming methods whereby around 75 per cent of commercial milk comes from pregnant cows (Qin *et al.*, 2004).

In a more recent study looking at the effects of persistent milk consumption beyond weaning (adults drinking milk) it was stated that epidemiological evidence points to increased dairy protein

consumption as a major dietary risk factor for the development of prostate cancer. This study reported how bioactive molecules in cow's milk initiate a signalling pathway (protein-mediated mTORC1 signalling) and that this, along with constant exposure to commercial cow's milk oestrogens derived from pregnant cows, may explain the observed association between high dairy consumption and increased risk of prostate cancer in Westernised societies. Normally, only infants consume milk up until weaning, so milk-mediated mTORC1 signalling is restricted to the postnatal growth phase of the vast majority of mammals – this is the natural state. Only milk proteins (compared to meat and fish) have the unique ability to preferentially increase both the insulin/IGF-1 and leucine signalling pathways necessary for maximal mTORC1 activation. In other words, the persistent consumption of cow's milk in humans provides a unique combination of factors that can lead to prostate cancer. The author suggests that a contemporary Palaeolithic diet and restriction of dairy protein intake may offer protection from the most common dairy-promoted cancer in men of Western societies (Melnik, *et al.*, 2012).

Numerous studies now indicate that the growth factor IGF-1 is associated with an increased risk of prostate cancer. In an early Swedish study, levels of IGF-1 were measured in blood samples from over 800 men, 281 of whom were later diagnosed as having prostate cancer. A strong correlation between

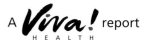

IGF-1 and prostate cancer was observed and it was concluded that circulating IGF-1 levels are associated with an increased risk for this disease (Stattin *et al.*, 2004). In a pooled reanalysis of worldwide prospective data based on 3,700 men with prostate cancer and 5,200 controls, researchers also concluded that high circulating IGF-1 concentrations are associated with a moderately increased risk for prostate cancer (Roddam *et al.*, 2008).

In 2007, an EPIC study (based on 630 cases and 630 controls), found a marginally increased prostate cancer risk for men with the highest IGF-1 levels (Allen *et al.*, 2007). In an extension of this work (this time based on 1,542 prostate cancer cases matched to 1,542 controls) IGF-1 concentration was significantly associated with an increased risk of prostate cancer. It was concluded that these results suggest that circulating concentrations of IGF-1 in middle to late adulthood are strongly associated with subsequent prostate cancer risk over the relatively long term (Price *et al.*, 2012). Campbell suggests that IGF-1 is turning out to be a predictor of certain cancers, including prostate cancer, in much the same way that cholesterol is a predictor of heart disease (Campbell and Campbell, 2005).

As stated previously the diet can influence IGF-1 levels in the blood and dairy products have been shown to increase the level of circulating IGF-1 (Young *et al.*, 2012). In a group of healthy, middle-aged men, dairy products, milk and calcium were all associated with raised IGF-1 levels (Gunnell *et al.*, 2003). In the same study, high intakes of vegetables and tomatoes, or tomato-containing products, were associated with lower levels of IGF-1. Furthermore, a study published in the *British Journal of Cancer* noted that vegan men had a nine per cent lower serum IGF-1 level than meat-eaters and vegetarians (Allen *et al.*, 2000). So again it is shown that milk increases IGF-1 and raised IGF-1 is linked to increased risk of cancer.

Research has clearly established that IGF-1 has a very important role in the development and progression of certain cancers, including prostate (Meinbach and Lokeshwar, 2006). Recent prospective epidemiological studies have also consistently shown strong associations between circulating IGF-1 levels and the subsequent risk of developing prostate cancer (Roddam *et al.*, 2008). Individuals with circulating IGF-1 levels at the upper end of the normal range are at significantly increased risk of subsequently developing prostate cancer years later.

Perhaps of greater significance though is the fact that recent evidence from population studies of prostate cancer suggests that the association with IGF-1 is not so much of an effect on cancer initiation, but reflects an effect on the risk of progression to clinically relevant disease (Holly 2013a). As mitogens (substances that encourage cell division), and antiapoptotic agents (substances that prevent apoptosis or cell death) IGF-1 may be important in carcinogenesis, possibly by increasing the risk of cellular transformation by enhancing cell turnover (Kucuk *et al.*, 2001). In other words, many men develop prostate cancer (or benign tumours) but IGF-1 may transform the tumours into a more aggressive form of cancer (Holly *et al.*, 2013a). Either way, IGF-1, from cow's milk, appears to be a risk factor that could easily be avoided by eliminating dairy foods from the diet.

It has been suggested that men with prostate cancer who increase consumption of plant-based foods and avoid dairy products and meat may significantly increase their chances of survival. Researchers from the Physicians Committee for Responsible Medicine (PCRM) reviewed eight observational studies and 17 intervention studies on the effect of a plant-based diet on prostate cancer results and found that a plant-based diet may slow prostate cancer progression and improve prognosis (Berkow *et al.*, 2007). They found that diets high in saturated fat are associated with a threefold higher risk of cancer progression and death, compared with a diet low in saturated fat. In addition, specific plant foods, including flaxseeds and lycopene-rich tomatoes, may help slow prostate cancer progression.

Possible mechanisms of action for lycopene, the major carotenoid in tomatoes, include the following:

- inhibition of growth in cancer cells by modulating the expression of cell cycle regulatory proteins
- modulation of the IGF-1/IGFBP-3 system (IGF signalling is thought to affect tissue growth and development with IGF-1 and IGF binding protein-3 (IGFBP-3) having putative pro- and anti-carcinogenic properties respectively)
- up-regulation of tumor suppressor proteins and increased gap junctional intercellular communication
- modulation of redox signaling
- prevention of oxidative DNA damage
- modulation of carcinogen metabolising enzymes

Source: Kucuk *et al.*, 2001.

While the precise molecular mechanisms underlying the development of prostate cancer are still being teased out, the effects of changing the diet have produced positive results. Researchers at the Preventative Medicine Research Institute in California evaluated the effects of dietary changes in 93 volunteers who had chosen not to undergo conventional treatment for early prostate cancer. This was a unique opportunity to observe the effects of diet and lifestyle changes without the confounding effects of radiation or surgery. Participants in the lifestyle-change group were placed on a vegan diet consisting primarily of fruits, vegetables, whole grains and pulses supplemented with soya, vitamins and minerals. Two standard tests were used to assess disease status. The first was a routine blood test measuring PSA levels; this protein produced by the prostate gland can be used to assess disease progression. The second test relied on differences in the growth rates of a human prostate cancer cells (LNCaP) treated with patient serum. This is a standard laboratory test used for evaluating the effects of conventional treatments of prostate cancer.

While none of the experimental (vegan) patients underwent conventional treatment during the study, six control patients underwent treatment due to an increase in PSA and/or progression of the disease on magnetic resonance imaging. PSA decreased four per cent in the experimental group but increased six per cent in the control group. Although the magnitude of these changes was relatively modest, the direction of change may be clinically significant since an increase in PSA predicts clinical progression in the majority of men with prostate cancer. In the second test, the growth of LNCaP prostate cancer cells was inhibited almost eight times more by serum from the experimental than from the control group. Changes in serum PSA and also in LNCaP cell growth were significantly associated with the degree of change in diet and lifestyle. It was concluded that intensive lifestyle changes may affect the progression of early, low grade prostate cancer (Ornish et al., 2005).

In the late 1980s, increasing the consumption of beans, lentils, peas, tomatoes, raisins, dates and other dried fruit was found to be associated with a significantly decreased risk of prostate cancer (Mills et al., 1989). A decade later, a study of over 47,000 men confirmed an inverse link between fructose and prostate cancer indicating that eating fruit offers some protection against prostate cancer (Giovannucci et al., 1998a). More recently, in a review of diet, lifestyle and prostate cancer it was observed that while meat and dairy are associated with an increased risk, the consumption of tomato products (which contain the antioxidant lycopene), vitamin E and selenium supplements have all been shown to decrease risk. Tomato ketchup is a source of lycopene and organic brands may contain up to three times as much lycopene as non-organic (Ishida and Chapman, 2004). A high level of physical activity was also identified as a factor decreasing the risk of prostate cancer (Wolk, 2005).

Studies have shown that the consumption of soya foods may be associated with a reduction in cancer risk in humans. In a meta-analysis of 15 epidemiologic studies on soya consumption and nine on isoflavones (the plant hormones in soya foods) in association with prostate cancer risk, results showed that soya foods are associated with a reduction in prostate cancer risk. This protection may be associated with the type and quantity of soy foods consumed (Yan and Spitznagel, 2009).

In summary, the data linking the consumption of cow's milk and dairy products to numerous different types of cancer provides a convincing argument for eliminating all animal foods from the diet while increasing the intake of whole grains, pulses (including soya), fruit and vegetables.

Colic

Colic was first mentioned in recorded history by the ancient Greeks (Cirgin Ellett, 2003), yet in 2013 the cause remains somewhat undetermined. Colic is the medical term for excessive, frequent crying in a baby who appears to be otherwise healthy and well fed. It is a poorly understood yet common condition that affects around one in five babies. However, the condition is not harmful and babies with colic continue to feed and gain weight normally. There is no evidence that colic has any long-term effects on a baby's health (NHS Choices, 2012i). A baby with colic may have several crying outbursts a day and this may occur a few times a week. The crying pattern usually begins within the first few weeks of life but often stops by the time the baby is four months old, by six months at the latest. Typically, a baby with colic will scream and draw up their legs, and may refuse to be comforted. It can be very distressing for parents, especially as the cause of colic remains largely unknown.

While the exact cause is unknown several factors are

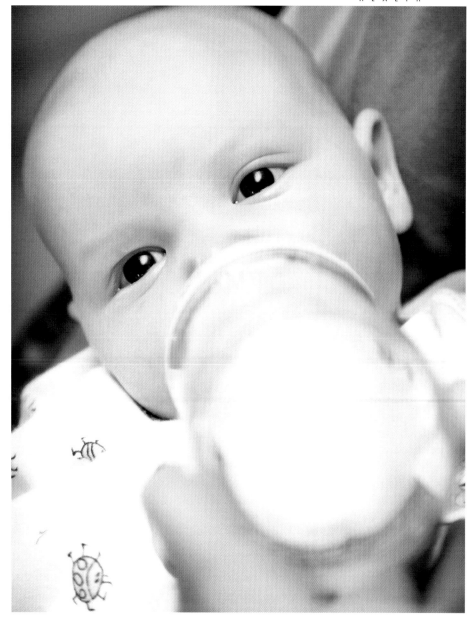

thought to contribute including poor digestion, lactose intolerance and/or a reaction to cow's milk proteins. Since the 1970s, numerous studies have indicated that certain components of cow's milk may lead to colic. In a clinical trial to investigate the effects of cow's milk whey proteins, 24 out of 27 infants with colic showed no symptoms of colic after whey protein was removed from their diet. In fact crying hours per day dropped from 5.6 hours to 0.7 hours (Lothe and Lindberg, 1989). In order to alleviate the negative effects of cow's milk whey proteins (and other milk proteins thought to cause colic) some infant formulas are hydrolysed, this means the proteins are broken up. These hydrolysed formulas are called hypoallergenic and have been shown to be effective in the treatment of colic in some infants (Lindberg, 1999; Jakobsson *et al.*, 2000; Lucassen *et al.*, 1998; Lucassen *et al.*, 2000).

Some differences in intestinal flora (the bacteria that inhabit the gut) have been identified in infants with colic (Lehtonen *et al.*, 1994; Savino *et al.*, 2004). Research suggests that altering intestinal flora might help prevent colic in formula-fed infants, who have well-known differences in gut flora compared to breast-fed infants (Newburg, 2000). Other reports that oligosaccharide (prebiotic) supplements in infant formulas may promote gastrointestinal health are inconclusive (Savino *et al.*, 2006). However, a formula specifically developed to simulate the beneficial effects of human breast milk and to reduce some of the common feeding problems of cow's milk formula-fed infants was tested in infants with colic. It contained partially hydrolysed whey proteins, a mixture of oligosaccharides (90 per cent galacto-oligosaccharides and 10 per cent fructo-oligosaccharides), low lactose, modified vegetable oil with 41 per cent of the palmitic acid in the beta-position and starch. In human milk,

palmitic acid is predominantly in the central or beta-position, whereas in cow's milk and infant formulas, it is mainly in the first and third position and may form calcium-fatty acid complexes which are poorly absorbed in the gut (Savino, 2006). In a previous observational study, within two weeks of feeding with this formula, a significant decrease in the number of colic episodes was observed in the majority of infants tested (Savino *et al.*, 2003). This study was performed to confirm the role of this new formula in infants with colic in a randomised prospective trial. Results showed that infants fed with the formula had a significant decrease in colic episodes after just one week of treatment compared to infants from the control group. The difference in crying time was even more significant after two weeks of treatment. This study provides compelling evidences for the relation between colic and type of feeding. However, the increasingly expensive and elaborate attempts to simulate human breast milk beg the question, why don't we put a more concerted effort into simply promoting breastfeeding?

In transient lactose intolerance, the enzyme lactase is not produced while there is illness in the gut, but is manufactured again once the gut has recovered. In a review investigating transient lactose intolerance as a cause of colic, a range of studies showed that crying time was reduced when formula or breast milk was incubated with the enzyme lactase (Buckley, 2000). It has been suggested that infant colic has a multiple aetiology; in other words, colic may be caused by a number of different factors including whey proteins, lactose and others.

The fact that the incidence of colic is similar in formula fed and breastfed infants has led scientists to investigate the role of the maternal diet in this condition and many reports now link the maternal intake of cow's milk to the occurrence of colic in exclusively breastfed infants. The breast milk of mothers who consume cow's milk and milk products has been shown to contain intact proteins from these foods. To test the possible role of cow's milk proteins in breast milk, researchers have investigated the effects of eliminating all dairy products from the mothers' diet. An early report linking cow's milk proteins in human breast milk to infantile colic date back to a letter published in the *Lancet* in the late 1970s (Jakobsson and Lindberg, 1978). The letter described how the symptoms of colic disappeared in 13 out of 19 infants whose mothers eliminated cow's milk from their diet. In a subsequent clinical trial designed by the same researchers, 66 breastfeeding mothers of infants with colic were put on a diet free from cow's milk. The colic disappeared in 35 of the infants and subsequently reappeared in 23 of them when cow's milk protein was reintroduced to the mothers' diet (Jakobsson and Lindberg, 1983). The authors suggest that a diet free of cow's milk may be useful as a first trial of treatment of infantile colic in breastfed infants.

Researchers at the Washington School of Medicine in Missouri US found that mothers of infants with colic had significantly higher levels of the cow's milk antibody immunoglobulin G (IgG) in their breast milk than mothers of infants without colic (Clyne and Kulczycki, 1991). The authors of this study suggest that bovine IgG present in breast milk may be involved in the development of colic. This link was confirmed more recently and again it was suggested that the maternal avoidance of milk and dairy products may be an effective treatment for colic in some breastfed infants (Estep and Kulczycki, 2000). A systematic review of nineteen studies and two literature reviews on medical and conventional interventions for infantile colic from 1980 to 2009 found some scientific evidence to support the use of a casein hydrolysate formula in formula-fed infants and a low-allergen maternal diet in breastfed infants with colic. However, they found little scientific evidence to support the use of lactase, additional fibre or behavioural interventions. They suggested that further research on low-allergenic formulas and maternal diets would be useful (Hall et al., 2012).

In a substantial review of 27 controlled trials published in the *British Medical Journal*, the elimination of cow's milk protein was deemed to be a highly effective treatment for infantile colic. The reviewers remained uncertain about the effectiveness of low lactose formula milks and the effectiveness of substitution with soya-based formula milks (although no adverse events were reported) while supporting the substitution of normal cow's milk formula for whey or casein protein hydrolysate (hypoallergenic) formulas, in which the milk protein is partially broken down to ease digestion (Lucassen, 1998).

Interestingly, Dr Benjamin Spock, author of the hugely popular book *Baby and Child* (over 50 million copies sold worldwide) warns that the proteins in cow's milk formulas can cause colic (Spock and Parker, 1998). Spock acknowledges that some infants that are allergic to cow's milk formula may be allergic to soya-based infant formula as well and that these infants are often given expensive hydrolysate formulas. However, he states that soya formulas have an important advantage over cow's milk formulas in that they contain none of the animal proteins linked with colic (and type 1 diabetes) and are free of lactose.

This said, it should be emphasised to parents who breastfeed, it is a good idea to continue breastfeeding as weaning on to formula milk may make the colic worse. If eliminating cow's milk and milk products from the maternal diet does not help, cutting out other foods may help. Researchers at the University of Minnesota tested a range of foods including cruciferous vegetables (cabbage, cauliflower, sprouts and broccoli) in an elimination diet in mothers of babies with colic. While the results showed that cow's milk had the strongest association with colic, other foods more weakly associated included: onions, chocolate, cabbage, broccoli and cauliflower (Lust et al., 1996).

In conclusion, colic is a common cause of maternal distress and family disturbance and more research is

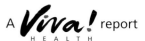
needed to develop solid evidence-based recommendations for successful treatment. However, eliminating cow's milk from the maternal diet (if breastfeeding) and avoiding cow's milk formula may help.

Constipation

Constipation is a condition in which bowel movements are infrequent or incomplete. While it is normal for some people to go to the toilet several times a day, others go less frequently. A change in the normal frequency of trips to the toilet can be an indicator of constipation. Similarly if you are going as frequently but having trouble passing stools, having to strain, this too may indicate constipation. Common symptoms include stomach ache and cramps, feeling bloated, nausea, a sense of fullness, headache, loss of appetite, fatigue and depression.

There are a number of factors that increase the risk of constipation, including:

- not eating enough fibre, such as fruit, vegetables and cereals
- a change in your routine or lifestyle, such as a change in your eating habits
- ignoring the urge to pass stools
- side effects of certain medication
- not drinking enough fluids
- anxiety or depression
- In children, poor diet, fear about using the toilet and poor toilet training can all be responsible

Source NHS Direct, 2012j.

In more detail, constipation may be caused by a range of factors including insufficient fluid in the diet, lack of fibre (fruit, vegetables and cereals) in the diet, lack of physical exercise, certain drugs (diuretics or painkillers, antidepressants and antacids that contain iron, calcium or aluminium), too much calcium or iron in the

diet, pregnancy, an excessive intake of tea or coffee (this increases urine production and so decreases the amount of fluid in the bowel). Other factors include surgery, haemorrhoids (piles) and psychological problems such as anxiety. Constipation may be a symptom of another medical condition such as irritable bowel syndrome (IBS).

The link between constipation and cow's milk intolerance was first made in medical literature in the 1950s (Clein, 1954). Since then, there have been numerous studies published confirming that this link exits. Researchers at the University of Palermo in Italy studied 65 children (aged from 11 to 72 months) suffering from chronic constipation (Iacono et al., 1998). All of these children had been treated with laxatives without success. After 15 days of observations (in a double-blind crossover study) each child received either cow's milk or soya milk for two weeks, and then had a week off when they could eat and drink anything they wanted. Then the feeding order was reversed, so that the group that had previously drunk cow's milk switched to soya and vice versa. The researchers (and children) were unaware of the order of treatment. Careful recordings of the bowel habits were made and a response to the treatment was defined as eight or more bowel movements during the two week treatment period. Results showed that 44 of the 65 children (68 per cent) had a response while receiving soya milk compared to none of the children receiving cow's milk. The results were most dramatic in children who had frequent runny noses, eczema or wheezing, which may have been a symptom of milk allergy in these children. Sometimes however, constipation can be the only symptom of cow's milk intolerance (or allergy).

In addition to cow's milk intolerance, cow's milk allergy in children can also cause chronic constipation. Some small-scale studies have observed how a cow's milk protein-free diet can alleviate constipation in children with cow's milk allergy (Daher et al.; 2001; Turunen, 2004). A larger randomised clinical study investigating the role of cow's milk allergy as a cause of chronic constipation in two groups of 70 children (aged 1-13) with chronic constipation compared the effects of a cow's milk free diet with cow's milk diet. All children had previously been treated with laxatives for at least three months without success. The test group received the cow's milk-free diet for four weeks. After that they received a cow's milk diet for two weeks. The control group received a cow's milk diet for the whole six weeks. After four weeks, 56 patients (80 per cent) of the test group had responded in comparison to 33 (47.1 per cent) patients in the control group. In the test group after two weeks challenge, 24 out of 56 responders (42.8 per cent) developed constipation again. 80 per cent of the constipated children tested positive for cow's milk allergy. The authors concluded that, in children, chronic constipation can be a symptom of cow's milk allergy and suggest that an elimination diet is advisable in all children with constipation unresponsive to laxative treatment (Dehghani et al., 2012).

Cow's milk protein-induced constipation in children is often associated with anal fissures (tears or ulcers that develops in the lining of the rectum or anus) and rectal eosinophilia (a condition in which abnormally high amounts of white blood cells called eosinophils are found in the gut lining. Eosinophilia occurs in a wide range of conditions including allergies such as asthma and cow's milk allergy). In children with cow's milk allergy, cow's milk may lead to painful defecation, perianal erythema or eczema and anal fissures with possible painful faecal retention, thus aggravating constipation (Andiran et al., 2003). For this particular symptom (constipation), it has been reported that tolerance of cow's milk may be achieved after an average of 12 months of strict avoidance (El-Hodhod et al., 2010). In other words, in children with cow's milk allergy-induced constipation, reintroducing cow's milk into the diet can trigger the constipation for an average time of up to one year. It is interesting that there is a persistent insistence on including a food in the diet that can cause such unpleasant and distressing symptoms when dairy food is not an essential component of the human diet.

Cow's milk may lead to constipation by two distinct modes of action: cow's milk intolerance or cow's milk allergy. In either case, studies suggest that cow's milk intolerance or allergy should be considered as a cause of constipation although the underlying mechanism still requires further investigation. In general it should be noted that dairy products supply children with unnecessary saturated fat while providing no dietary fibre whatsoever. Fibre is essential in the diet to maintain good bowel health through regular movements.

Coronary heart disease

Diseases of the heart and circulatory system are collectively called cardiovascular disease (CVD) and are a leading cause of death in the UK. Coronary heart disease (CHD) is one of the two main forms of CVD along with stroke. Over 1.6 million men and over one million women are affected by CHD. It is responsible for more than 88,000 deaths in the UK each year, an average of 224 people each day or one death every six minutes. Around one in six men and one in nine women die from CHD (BHF, 2013). Most deaths from CHD are caused by heart attacks. In the UK, there are about 124,000 heart attacks each year. There are also around 152,000 strokes in the UK each year, resulting in over 43,000 deaths (NHS Choices, 2012k).

CHD occurs when there is a build-up of fatty deposits (plaques) along the walls of the arteries that supply the heart with oxygenated blood. These plaques build up and clog the arteries making them narrower and restricting the blood flow. Blood clots can form at the site of a plaque in the coronary artery and cut off the blood supply to the heart. This can result in heart attack and sudden death. Like the heart (and other organs), the brain needs the oxygen provided by blood to function properly. If the supply of blood is restricted or stopped, a stroke may occur and brain cells could begin to die, it can lead to brain damage and possibly death. The plaques that block the arteries are made up of a fatty substance that contains cholesterol. Cholesterol is essential for cells but too much can lead to CHD and stroke. Lipoproteins carry cholesterol to and from the cells in the blood. Low-density lipoprotein (LDL) takes cholesterol from the liver to the cells, and high-density lipoprotein (HDL) carries excess cholesterol back to the liver for excretion. HDL is known as the 'good fat' while LDL ('bad fat') tends to build up on the walls of the arteries increasing the risk of CHD and stroke.

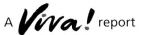

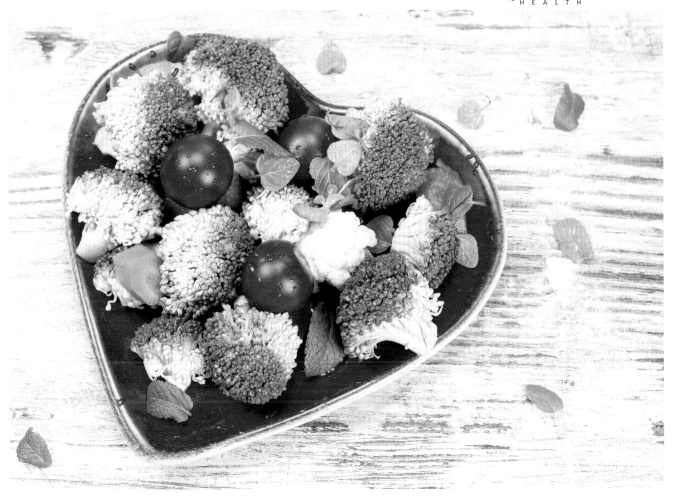

There are several well-documented risk factors for CVD including:

- **Smoking** – significantly increases the risk of CHD
- **Obesity** – more than a quarter of adults in England are obese and around 30 per cent of boys and girls aged two to 15 in England and Scotland are overweight or obese
- **Alcohol** – more than a third of men and over a quarter of women regularly exceed the government recommended level of alcohol intake
- **Blood pressure** – around one in three adults in England and Scotland have high blood pressure and nearly half of them are not receiving treatment for it
- **Cholesterol** – around six in 10 adults in England have cholesterol levels of 5mmol/l or above (you should aim to have a cholesterol level under 4mmol/l)
- **Poor diet** – less than one third of men and women currently eat the recommended five portions of fruit and vegetables per day in Britain, only around one in five boys and girls aged five to 15 consume the recommended amount

Source: BHF, 2013

Some risk factors put you at greater risk of CHD and stroke than others but the more risk factors you do have, the greater your chance of developing CVD. However, having a risk factor does not necessarily mean you will develop CVD, it just means it is more likely. So, limiting your risk factors reduces your risk.

Figure 7.0 Death rates from CHD for people aged 35-75 from 1968 to 2010.

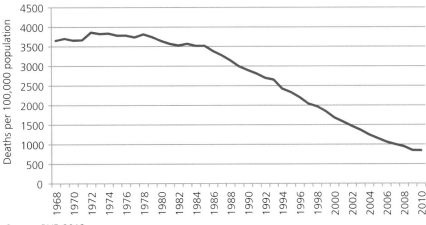

Source: BHF, 2012.

Figure 7.0 shows how the number of deaths from CHD has fallen markedly since the late 1960s. This is because of a combination of factors including improvements in medical treatment and lifestyle changes. For example a vast improvement has been made in the speed at which so-called clot-busting drugs are applied, which has had a huge impact in preventing death. Furthermore, nearly two million people receive drugs called statins that lower cholesterol levels and reduce the risk of heart disease. Research suggests that statins may prevent cardiovascular events and reduce subsequent mortality by up to 60 per cent (Mills *et al.*, 2008).

Many people have quit smoking, which has had a significant effect on lowering their risk of heart disease. Figures from the UK's Office of National Statistics' Opinions and Lifestyle Survey show that 45 per cent of adults smoked in 1974 compared with 20 per cent in 2012. This has contributed to the decline in smoking-related heart disease and subsequent mortality. The risk of CVD dramatically decreases when a person quits smoking and continues to fall rapidly for the first year and after five years the risk of CVD returns to the level of that of a non-smoker (Glantz and Gonzalez, 2012). UK Government initiatives encouraging people to reduce their salt intake (linked to high blood pressure) are also likely to have contributed to the decline in high blood pressure-related mortality (Office for National Statistics, 2013).

However, while fewer people are dying from CVD, the number of people living with it has remained relatively constant over the last decade. Figure 8.0 shows that from 2000 to 2010, the percentage of men and women (aged over 16 years) with CVD in Great Britain varied moderately, remaining between nine and 12 per cent (falling no lower than 9.4 and rising no higher than 11.9). The benefits we should be seeing, due to the advances in medical treatment and the reduction in smoking, are being negated by an increase in deaths attributable to rises in body mass index and diabetes.

Researchers from the Department of Applied Health Research, at the University College London used a well-known, tried and tested epidemiological model (IMPACT) to analyse the total population of England aged 25 and older in 2000 and 2007 (Bajekal *et al.*, 2012). They included all the major risk factors for CHD plus 45 current medical and surgical treatments in their model. They found that half (52 per cent) of the recent CHD mortality fall in England was attributable to improved treatment uptake. However, opposing trends in major lifestyle risk factors meant that the net contribution of these interventions amounted to only just over a third of the CHD deaths averted. In other words, despite the medical advances of the last ten years, plus the large drop in the number of smokers in the UK, we are not reaping the benefits as much as we could because of poor lifestyle and dietary choices. You could say it is a case of 'two steps forward and one step back'. Furthermore, concerns are that the decline in deaths from heart disease may be short lived due to the increasing levels of inactivity, the rise in obesity, the increase in cholesterol levels and the rise of type 2 diabetes.

The quest to identify dietary and lifestyle risk factors for CHD dates back over five decades. In 1946 Los Angeles physician Dr Lester Morrison began a study to determine the relationship of dietary fat intake to the incidence of CHD (Morrison, 1960). He reduced the dietary fat intake of 50 heart attack survivors and compared their health to 50 other heart attack survivors whose fat intake was left unchanged. After eight years, 38 of the control group had died compared to 22 of the low-fat group. After 12

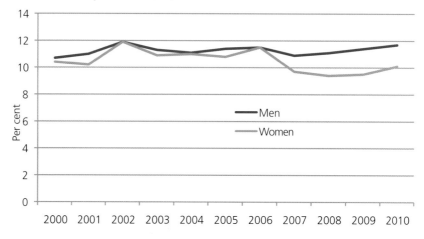

Figure 8.0 Prevalence of CVD in people aged over 16 in Great Britain, 2000-2010.

Source: BHF, 2012.

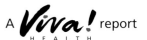

years, the entire control group had died but 19 of the low-fat diet group were still alive. Around the same time, the residents of Framingham, just outside Boston Massachusetts in the US, took part in a study to investigate the role of diet and lifestyle in CHD. The study began in 1948, and by observing who suffered from CHD and who did not, the Framingham Study established the concept of risk factors such as cholesterol, high blood pressure (hypertension), lack of physical exercise, smoking and obesity (Kannal *et al.*, 1961).

It is important to note that dietary risk factors for CVD do not just apply to adults. Various studies warn of the increased risk of CVD (later in life) associated with the consumption of cow's milk and cow's milk infant formula in young children. A review on infant feeding practices published in the US journal *Pediatrics* suggests that the consumption of whole milk should be discouraged in infants because of its potential role in atherosclerotic heart disease (Oski, 1985).

In 2002, a substantial report of a joint WHO/FAO expert consultation review of the evidence on the effects of diet and nutrition on chronic diseases stated that:

"Data from most, but not all, observational studies of term infants have generally suggested adverse effects of formula consumption on the other risk factors for cardiovascular disease (as well as blood pressure), but little information to support this finding is available from controlled clinical trials. Nevertheless, the weight of current evidence indicates adverse effects of formula milk on cardiovascular disease risk factors; this is consistent with the observations of increased mortality among older adults who were fed formula as infants. The risk for several chronic diseases of childhood and adolescence (e.g. type 1 diabetes, coeliac disease, some childhood cancers, inflammatory bowel disease) have also been associated with infant feeding on breast-milk substitutes and short-term breastfeeding" (WHO/FAO, 2002).

A more recent review of the current literature concurred that being breastfed as an infant (as opposed to cow's milk formula-feeding) is associated with a reduction in blood pressure, cholesterol and a lower risk of obesity and diabetes in adult life. The authors stated that although the effects on CVD risk

factors are modest, breastfeeding rates are suboptimal in many countries and strategies to promote breastfeeding could therefore confer important benefits for cardiovascular health at a population level (Robinson and Hall, 2012). The authors concluded that there is a growing recognition of the need for a life course approach to understanding how adult diseases, such as CVD, develop and there is now significant evidence that links patterns of infant feeding to different health outcomes both in the short and longer term.

As stated, a number of risk factors are now firmly associated with CHD including high cholesterol levels, high blood pressure, family history of heart disease, diabetes, obesity and smoking. Additionally, there is much evidence linking CHD to poor dietary practices, including the high consumption of saturated fats, salt and refined carbohydrates, and the low consumption of fruits and vegetables (WHO/FAO, 2002).

A certain amount of cholesterol is essential for good health, but high cholesterol levels in the blood are associated with an increased risk of CHD and stroke. This is because cholesterol contributes towards the build-up of fatty plaques on the artery walls which results in the narrowing of the arteries and can lead to a blockage and subsequent failure or death of the organ that the artery provides blood to. The organs affected often include the heart (heart attack) and brain (stroke), but may affect other organs such as the kidneys (kidney failure). But what determines blood cholesterol levels? Contrary to popular belief, most of our cholesterol does not come from the diet but is produced within the body by the liver. Only a small amount of our cholesterol (estimates vary from 15 to 20 per cent) comes from the diet. Cholesterol is found only in animal foods and is particularly concentrated in eggs and organ meats. Even high-fat plant foods, such as avocados, nuts and seeds, contain no cholesterol whatsoever, so a plant-based vegan diet is cholesterol-free. We have no actual dietary requirement for cholesterol, in other words we do not need to eat foods that contain cholesterol as the liver can manufacture as much as is required. However, there is no mechanism limiting the amount of cholesterol produced by the liver and cholesterol production can rise to unhealthy levels.

So what causes high cholesterol production in the liver? The answer lies in the types of foods we eat: diets high in animal protein and saturated animal fats have been shown to increase cholesterol. The cholesterol-raising effects of saturated fat are well-documented. In a review of the literature, researchers from the Department of Nutrition at the Harvard School of Public Health in Boston, Massachusetts, found compelling evidence that the types of fat are more important than total amount of fat in determining the risk of CHD (Hu *et al.*, 2001). Here the culprit is saturated fat, and controlled clinical trials have shown that replacing this type of fat with polyunsaturated fat is more effective in lowering cholesterol and reducing the risk of CHD than reducing total fat consumption. In 1985, research published in the *Journal of the American Medical Association* suggested that dairy products are a major source of dietary saturated fat and cholesterol and that ingestion of high-fat dairy products raises both total and LDL 'bad' cholesterol levels (Sacks *et al.*, 1985). It is now widely accepted that diets high in animal fats are unhealthy and that reducing the saturated fat intake is very important for reducing the risk of CHD. The UK Government recommends avoiding or cutting down on fatty foods. Foods high in saturated fat include: meat pies, sausages and fatty cuts of meat, butter, ghee, lard, cream, hard cheese, cakes and biscuits and foods containing coconut or palm oil (NHS Choices, 2013c). Like saturated fats, trans fats can also raise cholesterol levels. Trans fats are found naturally at low levels in meat and dairy products and foods containing hydrogenated vegetable oil, including processed foods such as biscuits, cakes, fast food, pastry, margarines and spreads. However, most people in the UK don't eat a lot of trans fats as many supermarkets in the UK have removed hydrogenated vegetable oil from their products.

As stated, replacing saturated fat with polyunsaturated fat is more effective in lowering cholesterol and reducing the risk of CHD than reducing

total fat consumption. Studies on the protective effect of seafood polyunsaturated omega-3 fatty acids (EPA and DHA) have produced mixed results because of the relatively high levels of pollutants found in oily fish. A 2012 meta-analysis published in the *Journal of the American Medical Association* of 20 studies and 68,680 patients found that fish oil supplementation did not reduce the chance of death, cardiac death, heart attack or stroke (Rizos *et al.*, 2012). Furthermore, some positive results have been wildly exaggerated (NHS Choices, 2012l). In a meta-analysis of studies looking at the plant-based omega-3 fatty acid ALA (found in soya beans, walnuts and canola/rapeseed oil) it was found that each gram per day increment of ALA intake was associated with a 10 per cent lower risk of CHD

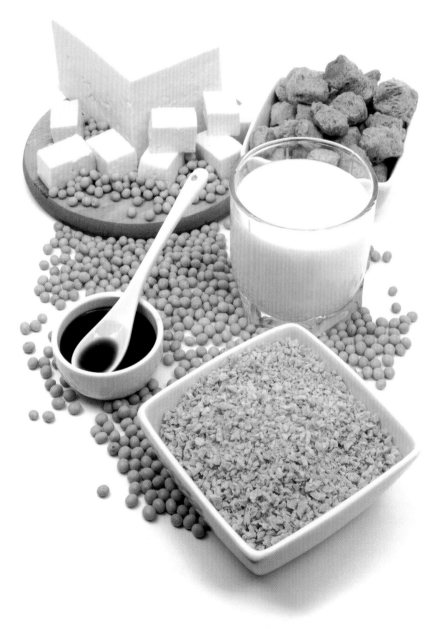

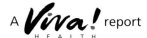

death (Pan *et al.*, 2012). The authors state that compared with seafood omega-3 fatty acids, ALA from plant sources is more affordable and widely available globally. Thus, whether ALA can reduce the risk of CVD is of considerable public health importance. It should be noted that algal sources of EPA and DHA are now available in supplement form for people concerned about their omega-3 intake.

In *The China Study*, Campbell observes that animal protein intake correlates directly with heart disease incidence, which he attributes to the cholesterol-raising effect of animal protein. Conversely, Campbell notes that eating plant protein lowers cholesterol (Campbell and Campbell, 2005). Studies have shown that replacing animal milk protein (casein) with soya protein reduces blood cholesterol, even when the fat intake remains unchanged (Lovati *et al.*, 1987; Sirtori *et al.*, 1999). Exactly how soya protein lowers cholesterol is uncertain, although a range of theories have been proposed. One hypothesis suggests that the amino acid composition of soya protein causes changes in cholesterol metabolism (possibly via the endocrine system). Others propose that non-protein components (such as saponins, fibre, phytic acid, minerals and isoflavones) associated with soya protein affect cholesterol metabolism either directly or indirectly (Potter, 1995). The most popular theory currently accepted is that soya protein reduces cholesterol metabolism in the liver by increasing the removal of LDL 'bad' cholesterol. The precise mechanism is thought to involve enhanced LDL-degradation by increased binding of LDL to receptors (Sirtori *et al.*, 1977; Lovati *et al.*, 2000).

A cross-sectional study of 1,033 pre- and postmenopausal women selected from the Oxford arm of the EPIC study (including 361 non-vegetarians, 570 vegetarians and 102 vegans) found that soya protein intake was inversely associated with total and LDL cholesterol levels. LDL ('bad') cholesterol in women with a soya protein intake of at least six grams per day was 12.4 per cent lower than that in women who consumed less than 0.5 grams per day (Rosell *et al.*, 2004).

More recently, a meta-analysis of studies examining the extent to which soya foods could reduce LDL cholesterol found that replacing meat or dairy protein with 13 grams of soya protein resulted in a LDL cholesterol reduction of 0.15mmol/l, 50 grams of soya protein reduced the level by 0.25mmol/l (Jenkins *et al.*, 2010). This represents a reduction of

around 4.3 per cent in LDL cholesterol with a potential additional reduction of 3.6-6.0 per cent due to displacement of saturated fat and cholesterol depending on the diet and the foods displaced. Based on these assumptions, the authors concluded that soya foods have the potential to lower LDL cholesterol by as much as 10.3 per cent. The authors state that the displacement value may be unique to soya, because other cholesterol-lowering foods are added to the diet rather than exchanged for suboptimal (meat and dairy) foods. They say that this makes soya a particularly valuable tool in the dietary armamentarium to reduce serum cholesterol. In addition, many soya products could be beneficial to cardiovascular and overall health because of their high content of polyunsaturated fats, fibre, vitamins and minerals and low content of saturated fat. Replacing cheese, meat and other animal foods with soya can mean using tofu, soya beans (edamame) or soya milk (in a white sauce). Soya-based faux meats (such as soya mince) can be used although the amount of processed food in the diet should be limited as they can contain relatively high levels of saturated fat and salt, but still remain a healthier option than meat and dairy.

Many other plant foods (and components of them) are known to possess cholesterol-lowering properties including nuts, plant sterols and viscous (soluble) fibres. Individually, these plant food components can be expected to lower LDL cholesterol in the range of 3-10 per cent, far less than the 40-60 per cent reductions achievable with statins. However, collectively they could reduce LDL cholesterol by up to 30 per cent, which would have a considerable impact on preventing CHD (Jenkins *et al.*, 2010).

Eating a diet that contains plenty of soluble fibre can help to reduce the amount of cholesterol in the blood and so reduce the risk of CHD. Good sources of soluble fibre include oats, beans, peas, lentils, chick peas, fruit and vegetables (NHS Choices, 2013c). Increased consumption of fruit and vegetables is associated with a reduced risk of CHD. A meta-analysis of twelve cohort studies including 278,459 individuals (9,143 CHD events) with an average follow-up of 11 years found that, increasing consumption of fruit and vegetables from less than three to more than five servings per day reduced CHD risk by 17 per cent. The authors state that these results provide strong support for the recommendations to consume more than five servings of fruit and vegetables a day (He *et al.*, 2007). The government recommend that we eat at least five portions of fruit and vegetables each day.

Dr Dean Ornish, best known for his Lifestyle Heart Trial, investigated the role of a low-fat, high-fibre diet coupled to lifestyle changes in heart disease patients. Ornish treated 28 heart disease patients with diet and lifestyle changes alone. They followed a low-fat plant-based diet including unrestricted amounts of fruits, vegetables and grains. They also practised stress management techniques and exercised regularly. After one year 82 per cent of the test group experienced regression of their heart disease, including a 91 per cent reduction in the frequency of heart pain compared to 165 per cent increase in the control group (Ornish *et al.*, 1990). No conventional drug or surgery related therapies compare with these results (Campbell and Campbell, 2005).

A study published in the *Journal of the American College of Nutrition* investigating the risk factors associated with CHD found that African-American vegans exhibit a more favourable serum lipid profile (a healthier balance of fats in the blood) compared to vegetarians who ate milk, milk products and eggs (Toohey *et al.*, 1998). This means that the vegans had healthier levels of total cholesterol, LDL and HDL in their blood compared to the vegetarians. The major factors contributing to this result were thought to be the lower saturated fat intake and higher fibre intake of vegans.

Examining the incidence of CHD in other cultures allows us to draw conclusions about the role of diet in disease. Several studies have shown that certified death rates from CHD are linked country-by-country with milk consumption (Moss and Freed, 2003). In The China Study, Campbell was astonished at the low rates of CHD in the southwest Chinese provinces of Sichuan and Guizhou; between 1973 and 1975 not one single person died of CHD before the age of 64 among 246,000 men and 181,000 women (Campbell and Campbell, 2005). Campbell suggests these figures reflect the important protective role of low blood cholesterol levels observed in rural China.

A joint report between the Medical Research Council and the British Heart Foundation states that the average blood total cholesterol level for people aged 16 and above in the UK is about 5.5mmol/l. In China (where there is much less heart disease), mean total cholesterol levels in the cities are about 4.5mmol/l for men and women aged 35-64, and levels in the countryside are even lower (MRC/BHF, 2006). According to the WHO, almost a fifth (18 per cent) of global stroke events and about 56 per cent of global heart disease is attributable to total

cholesterol levels above 3.2mmol/l (WHO, 2003). It could be argued that genetic differences between races may affect the risk factors for CHD and other diseases. However, Campbell's observations that Japanese men in Hawaii and California have much higher levels of blood cholesterol and incidence of CHD than Japanese men in Japan confirms that some risk factors are environmental rather than genetic. In other words, the choices we make about the food we eat and how we live can have a significant impact on heart health.

Since the early 1990s the amino acid homocysteine has become the subject of much interest among the scientific community. Evidence suggests that homocysteine damages the lining of blood vessels and enhances blood clotting. Elevated concentrations of homocysteine in the blood have been linked to an increased risk for both heart disease and stroke. Homocysteine is converted into the amino acid methionine in the presence of vitamin B12. In the same reaction, methyltetrahydrofolate is converted to folate which is used in the synthesis of DNA. This entire reaction relies on sufficient supplies of vitamins B6, B12 and folate. In B12 deficiency, the amount of homocysteine in the body can escalate to potentially dangerous levels and has been linked to a range of disorders including depression, dementia, damage to the inner lining of the artery walls and may be a trigger for CHD. While increased homocysteine levels have been observed in some vegetarians and vegans they do not occur in those ensuring an adequate B12 intake of three micrograms per day, whereas elevated homocysteine levels are not uncommon among meat-eaters due to a low folate intake (Walsh, 2003). Additionally, elevated serum homocysteine levels tend to increase in the elderly as incidence of B12 deficiency occurs more frequently. Interestingly, a recent study showed how a daily serving of breakfast cereal fortified with folic acid, B6 and B12 not only contributed to the plasma status of these vitamins but significantly reduced homocysteine concentrations in a randomly selected group of relatively healthy 50-85 year olds (Tucker *et al.*, 2004).

The role of a vegetarian and vegan diet in nutrition and health was examined among a large group of vegetarians in the Oxford Vegetarian Study (Appleby *et al.*, 1999). This was a prospective study of 6,000 vegetarians and 5,000 non-vegetarian controlled subjects recruited in the UK between 1980 and 1984. In this study vegans had lower cholesterol

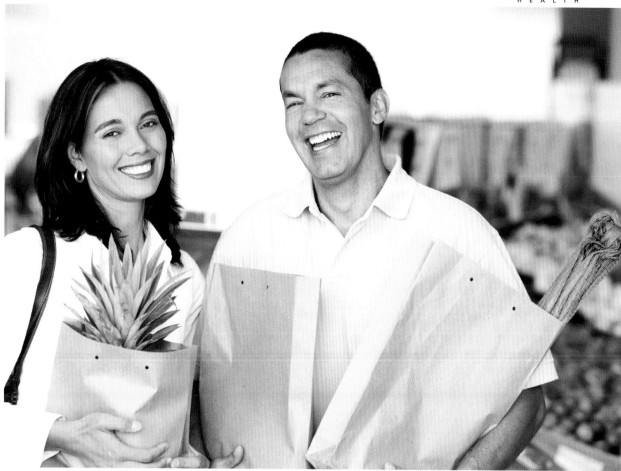

levels than meat-eaters (vegetarians and fish-eaters had intermediate or similar values). Meat and cheese consumption were positively associated, and dietary fibre intake was inversely associated, with cholesterol levels. After 12 years of follow-up, mortality from heart disease was positively associated with estimated intakes of total animal fat, saturated animal fat and dietary cholesterol. A subsequent review of the literature comparing the health of Western vegetarians to non-vegetarians found that vegetarians had lower cholesterol levels (by about 0.5mmol/l) and a lower mortality from heart disease (by about 25 per cent). It was suggested that **the widespread adoption of a vegetarian diet could prevent approximately 40,000 deaths from heart disease in Britain each year** (Key *et al.*, 1999).

Taken together, the evidence shows that a plant-based diet reduces the risk of CHD. This may be for a range of reasons including the cholesterol-lowering effect of fibre. It has been suggested that the antioxidants (beta-carotene and vitamins C and E) contained in fruit and vegetables and cereals prevent saturated fats from being converted into cholesterol in your body. Whatever the precise mechanism, the evidence is clear: a plant-based diet containing plenty of fruits and vegetables and whole grains reduces the risk of CHD. There is much speculation about how the consumption of animal foods increases the risk of CHD. Again, the precise mechanisms involved may be unresolved, but it is clear that the more animal foods a person eats, the

higher their risk. In summary, animal protein and saturated animals fats increase blood cholesterol and the risk of CHD while plant protein and fibre lowers cholesterol and reduces the risk. Therefore, to reduce the risk of CHD we should reduce the amount of animal foods in the diet and eat more wholegrain, plant-based foods.

There are of course other factors that can contribute to the risk of CHD. Exercise is extremely important as it increases HDL cholesterol levels, which in turn helps keep LDL cholesterol levels down. Exercise also helps control weight. As stated, smoking is a major risk factor of CHD as it hardens the arteries, causing them to narrow. Alcohol consumption can increase the risk so it should be limited and binge drinking avoided.

Crohn's disease

Crohn's disease is a chronic inflammatory bowel disease (IBD). It is a long-term condition that causes inflammation of the lining of the digestive system. The symptoms are similar to other bowel conditions such as irritable bowel syndrome (IBS) and another IBD ulcerative colitis. Crohn's disease commonly occurs in the ileum (the lower part of the small intestine), but it can affect any part of the bowel. In fact it can occur anywhere along the entire alimentary tract from the mouth to the anus. In most cases though, Crohn's disease occurs in sections of the bowel which become inflamed, ulcerated and

thickened. Symptoms can include diarrhoea, abdominal pain, fatigue (extreme tiredness), unintended weight loss and blood and mucus in the faeces (NHS Choices, 2013d). There may be long periods lasting for weeks or months where there are mild or even no symptoms, this is known as remission. Remission may be followed by periods where symptoms are particularly disruptive and/or distressing, these are known as flare-ups.

According to the National Association for Colitis and Crohn's Disease, the disease affects about one in every 1,000 people in the UK (NACC, 2010). There are currently at least 115,000 people living with Crohn's disease in the UK. It can affect people of all ages, including children but most cases first develop between the ages of 16 and 30. A large number of cases also develop between the ages of 60 and 80. It affects slightly more women than men, but in children more boys are affected than girls. Crohn's disease is more common in white people than in black or Asian people. It is most prevalent among Jewish people of European descent (NHS Choices, 2013e). Over time, inflammation may damage parts of the digestive system, resulting in additional complications, such as stricture (narrowing of the intestine) and fistula (a channel that develops between the anal canal and the skin near the anus). These problems usually require surgical treatment. The condition can lead to delay of growth and puberty in children, as well as affecting fertility and sexual relationships in adults (NICE, 2012).

There is currently no cure for Crohn's disease so the aims of treatment are to stop inflammation, relieve symptoms, induce and maintain remission and avoid surgery wherever possible. In the last decade, there have been a number of new drugs licensed for the condition; glucocorticosteroids can be

offered to induce remission and azathioprine or mercaptopurine can be offered as maintenance treatment (NICE, 2012). The National Institute for Health and Care Excellence (NICE) guidance suggests that the first treatment offered to reduce symptoms is usually corticosteroids (steroid medication). If this doesn't help, immunosuppressants (medication to suppress the immune system) and medication to reduce inflammation may be used. In some cases, surgery may be required to remove the inflamed section of the intestine. Once the symptoms under control, further medication may be used to help maintain remission.

Although the exact cause of Crohn's disease remains unclear, research suggests that a combination of factors may be responsible including:

• **Genetics** – genes that you inherit from your parents may increase your risk of developing Crohn's disease

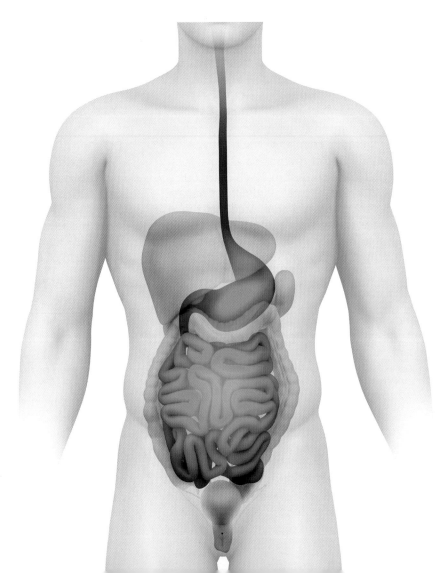

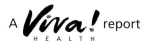
- **The immune system** – the inflammation may be caused by a problem with the immune system (the body's defence against infection and illness) that causes it to attack healthy bacteria in the gut
- **Previous infection** – a previous infection may trigger an abnormal response from the immune system
- **Smoking** – smokers with Crohn's disease usually have more severe symptoms than non-smokers
- **Environmental factors** – Crohn's disease is most common in westernised countries, such as the UK, and least common in poorer parts of the world, such as Africa, which suggests the environment (particularly sanitation) has a part to play

Source: NHS Choices, 2013d.

It has been proposed that an environmental factor leading to Crohn's disease is a pathogenic bacterium. The most popular candidate is the infectious bacterium *Mycobacterium avium* subspecies *paratuberculosis* (MAP). MAP infection is widespread in domestic livestock and is present in retail pasteurised cow's milk in the UK and potentially elsewhere and water supplies are also at risk (Bull *et al.*, 2003). The overall prevalence of MAP infection in US dairy herds was reported by a USDA survey (1991-2007) to be 68.1 per cent and it is suggested that MAP infection in farmed animals is also widespread in many areas of Western Europe and elsewhere (Hermon-Taylor, 2009). As MAP contaminates and persists in natural watercourses and the environment, it is found in dairy products, it can survive milk pasteurisation and it is present in meat from infected animals and there are concerns that water supplies may be contaminated, it is inevitable that human populations are widely exposed. MAP is a robust and versatile pathogen which has been shown to cause chronic inflammation in the intestines of many species of animal, including primates. MAP causes a chronic gastrointestinal infection called Johne's disease in cattle and other ruminants. The rising incidence of Crohn's disease reported from several former low incidence countries in Asia shows that, as with Johne's disease, Crohn's disease is spreading worldwide (Hermon-Taylor *et al.*, 2009).

A substantial body of evidence supports the causal link between MAP and Crohn's disease. Researchers at the University of Wisconsin used a range of modern molecular techniques to search for and confirm the presence of MAP in patients with IBDs including Crohn's. The results showed MAP was present in around 20 per cent of Crohn's patients compared to less than seven per cent of controls (without Crohn's). Although these results did not provide the substantive evidence initially anticipated the researchers concluded that MAP (or some similar species) infects a subset of IBD patients (Collins *et al.*, 2000). In another study, Professor John Hermon-Taylor and colleagues at St George's Hospital Medical School in London tested a group of patients with and without Crohn's disease for MAP. Using improved molecular biology techniques that increased the sensitivity of the tests, this time 92 per cent of patients with Crohn's disease tested positive compared to 26 per cent of the controls. These patients were from the UK, Ireland, US, Germany and United Arab Emirates, suggesting exposure to this pathogen occurs on an international basis. They concluded that the discovery that MAP is present in the majority of Crohn's patients would suggest a causal link between this bacterium and the condition (Bull *et al.*, 2003). Since then, additional reports have confirmed MAP as a predominant feature of Crohn's disease (Autschbach *et al.*, 2005; Sechi *et al.*, 2005). MAP can be notoriously difficult to detect in humans but when validated methodologies have been used, most people with Crohn's disease have been found to be infected with MAP (Hermon-Taylor *et al.*, 2009).

But how does MAP infection occur? The answer may lie under our very noses, depending on what we are drinking. MAP can survive the pasteurisation process, indeed an FSA-commissioned survey in 2002 found MAP in two per cent of pasteurised milk on sale in the UK (FSA, 2002a). However, researchers from the Department of Surgery at St George's Hospital Medical School in London detected MAP in 22 of 312 (seven per cent) of samples of whole pasteurised cow's milk obtained from retail outlets throughout central and southern England from September 1991 to March 1993. Alarmingly this study revealed the presence of peak periods in January to March and in September to November, when up to 25 per cent of samples tested positive for MAP (Millar *et al.*, 1996). Taken together with data on the prevalence of MAP infection in herds in the UK, the known secretion of MAP in milk from infected animals and the inability of laboratory conditions simulating pasteurisation to ensure the killing of all these slow-growing organisms, the authors of this study concluded that there is a high risk, particularly at peak times, that residual MAP will be present in retail pasteurised cow's milk in England.

In response to concerns about the presence of MAP in retail milk, the FSA devised a strategy to control MAP in milk at all stages of the food chain (FSA, 2003). This strategy aims to ensure hygienic milking practices and effective pasteurisation of milk and reduce the level of MAP in dairy herds. Of course the overall aim is to reduce the likelihood of consumers being exposed to MAP. However, this strategy does not consider alternative routes of exposure. In 2006 the strategy was reviewed and FSA Board Members were informed of progress, provided with an update on developments and told that no action was required. The report concluded "the Agency is not aware of any developments to suggest that its current advice on the drinking of milk needs updating at this time. The Agency and DH [The Department of Health], together with their expert committees, continue to keep evidence on the possible link between MAP and Crohn's disease under review" (FSA, 2006).

MAP is a robust organism which can survive for months or even years in the environment which is a cause of much concern as infected animals excrete huge numbers of MAP in their faeces. In South Wales, researchers sampled river water from the Taff which runs off the hills and through the city of Cardiff and detected MAP in 32.3 per cent of the samples (Pickup et al., 2005). The hills are grazed by livestock in which MAP is endemic. Previous research in Cardiff has shown a steep increase in the incidence of Crohn's disease. Given that inhalation is a probable route of MAP infection in cattle, it was suggested that the pattern of clustering of Crohn's disease in Cardiff may be due to people inhaling aerosols carrying MAP from the river. Other locations around the world, with similar geographic characteristics to the landscape in Cardiff, have since been identified as having higher rates of Crohn's disease. In New Zealand, a high incidence of Crohn's disease has been reported in the Canterbury region of South Island where Christchurch is the principal city. Rivers run from the mountains in the northwest across rich agricultural pastures and then around either side of Christchurch before entering the sea. A small river meanders through the city itself. As stated, these features resemble the situation in Cardiff. Similarly, a higher incidence of Crohn's disease has been observed in the US, in Winnipeg, Minnesota. The city straddles the junction of two large rivers; the Red River and the Assiniboine River. The 'hot spot' of Crohn's disease in Winnipeg is probably due to local exposure to high levels of waterborne MAP brought down from the

agricultural river catchments of the US Midwest, meeting those from the provinces of Manitoba, Saskatchewan and Alberta (Hermon-Taylor, 2009). Avoiding dairy products alone may not be enough to ensure avoiding exposure to MAP, although if everyone reduced their intake of animal products there would be fewer cattle and therefore less MAP present in the environment.

Some evidence from clinical trials suggests that anti-MAP treatment may be able to heal Crohn's disease in some people. When anti-MAP treatment works in so-called 'responders' receiving treatment with drug combinations (including rifabutin and clarithromycin) the clinical and pathological improvements can be dramatic. Furthermore, some of the clinical benefit resulting from treatment with immunosuppressants (such as mercaptopurine or methotrexate) may actually be a consequence of their anti-MAP action. However, MAP infections are difficult to eradicate, the organisms are generally resistant to drugs conventionally used in the treatment of tuberculosis (Hermon-Taylor, 2009).

The hypothesis that MAP causes Crohn's disease remains controversial and is disputed by some. Professor Ryan Balfour Sartor, from the Department of Medicine at the University of North Carolina in the US says that we must determine whether MAP infection causes human disease or whether this environmental contaminant innocently lodges in ulcerated mucosa. He asks if MAP might be analogous to *Helicobacter pylori* in peptic ulcer disease, gastritis and gastric cancer, where host genetics and microbial virulence factors determine immune responses that mediate clinical disease in a small minority of patients exposed to a widespread infectious agent. He says that this controversy has persisted far too long and needs to be resolved (Sartor, 2005).

For patients that have developed Crohn's disease avoiding foods that precipitate the symptoms has proved to be a successful way of avoiding drug (corticosteroid) therapy. In the *Lancet* in 1993, researchers from a Cambridge hospital reported that altering the diet was as effective in producing remission of Crohn's disease as corticosteroid treatment thus providing an alternative therapeutic strategy to treating Crohn's. The research showed that the food intolerances were predominantly to cereals, dairy products and yeast (Riordan et al., 1993). The foods that trigger symptoms differ for each person with Crohn's disease and no single diet

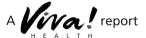
has been established to alleviate the symptoms. Types of food and drink that have been associated with worsening symptoms include:

* Milk and dairy products
* Alcohol
* Spicy foods
* Fatty foods
* High-fibre foods

Source: NHS Direct Wales, 2013.

Not all patients respond equally to dietary changes, many simply remove symptom-provoking foods that affect them, such as dairy, wheat, corn and certain fruits and vegetables (Brown and Roy, 2010). In a review of the evidence coupled to existing dietary information provided patient-centred IBD-related organisations, scientists from the Department of Complementary and Alternative Medicine at John A Burns School of Medicine at the University of Hawaii in Manoa are attempting to create new 'global

practice guidelines' that will consolidate the existing information regarding diet and IBD. They include nutritional deficiency screening, avoiding foods that worsen symptoms, eating smaller meals at more frequent intervals, drinking adequate fluids, avoiding caffeine and alcohol, taking vitamin/mineral supplements, eliminating dairy if lactose intolerant, limiting excess fat, reducing carbohydrates and reducing high-fibre foods during flare ups. They say that mixed advice exists regarding probiotics and note that enteral nutrition (the delivery of nutritionally complete food directly into the stomach) is recommended for Crohn's disease patients in Japan, which differs from practices in the USA and UK (Brown *et al.*, 2011). Manipulating the diet rather than relying on drug therapy may be particularly important as corticosteroid treatment in patients with Crohn's disease has been linked to osteoporosis (Dear *et al.*, 2001).

Stress and smoking can also influence the course of Crohn's disease.

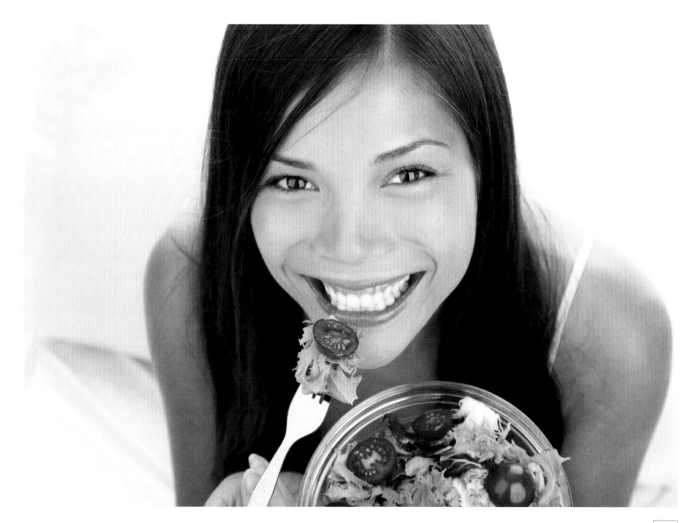

Diabetes

Diabetes mellitus is a chronic disease caused by too much sugar (glucose) in the blood. Blood sugar levels rise when there is not enough insulin in the blood, or the insulin that is in the blood does not work properly. Insulin is an important hormone secreted by the beta cells of the islets of Langerhans in the pancreas. It regulates blood sugar levels by, for example, promoting the uptake of glucose into the cells. When things go wrong, high levels of glucose in the blood can cause damage to the nerves and blood vessels. Without treatment diabetes can lead to long-term health problems including kidney failure, gangrene, sensory loss, ulceration, blindness, cardiovascular disease and stroke.

There are two main types of diabetes; type 1 and type 2. A third type of diabetes, gestational diabetes, develops in some women during pregnancy but usually disappears after giving birth.

Type 1 (insulin-dependent diabetes) occurs when the body produces little or no insulin. People who have type 1 diabetes must check the levels of glucose in their blood regularly and will need treatment for the rest of their lives. Type 1 diabetes is sometimes called juvenile-onset diabetes because it tends to develop before the age of 40, often in the teenage years. The peak age for diagnosis in the UK is between 10 and 14 years but is becoming younger with a steep rise in the under-fives (Williams and Pickup, 2004). Over the past 60 years, the worldwide incidence of type 1 diabetes has been increasing by 3-5 per cent per year, doubling approximately every 20 years with a rapid increase in the number of very young children affected (TEDDY Study Group, 2008). Symptoms include a frequent urge to urinate, extreme thirst and hunger, weight loss, fatigue, irritability and nausea. The cause of type 1 diabetes is poorly understood, but evidence suggests it involves a combination of genetic

factors and environmental triggers. Type 1 diabetes is usually treated with regular injections of insulin to regulate blood sugar levels.

Type 2 diabetes occurs either when the body does not produce enough insulin or when it cannot use the insulin produced. This type of diabetes is linked with obesity. If you are overweight or obese (you have a body mass index of 30 or more), you are at greater risk of developing type 2 diabetes. In particular, fat around your abdomen (tummy) puts you at increased risk because it releases chemicals that can upset the body's cardiovascular and metabolic systems (NHS Choices, 2012m). Type 2 diabetes occurs mostly in people over the age of 40, but is now increasingly affecting people at a much younger age.

The main symptoms are common to both types of diabetes: feeling very thirsty, urinating frequently, particularly at night, feeling very tired and weight loss with loss of muscle bulk. Other symptoms of type 2 diabetes include: itchiness around the vagina or penis, or regular bouts of thrush (a yeast infection), blurred vision that is caused by the lens of your eye becoming very dry, cramps, constipation and skin infections. Not all symptoms occur and those that do might be subtle and may go unnoticed for years. Blood sugar levels in type 2 diabetes can be controlled by lifestyle changes including regular exercise coupled to diet control and weight loss.

Type 1 diabetes is an autoimmune disease where the immune system's 'soldiers', known as T-cells, destroy the body's own insulin-producing beta cells in the pancreas. This type of response is thought to involve a genetic predisposition (diabetes in the family) coupled to an environmental trigger.

In the UK, about 90 per cent of all adults with diabetes have type 2 diabetes. While rising obesity levels have contributed to

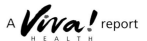

the increase in the incidence of type 2 diabetes, the increase in obesity does not explain the huge increase in the number of cases of type 1 diabetes seen over the last few decades. The number of under-fives with Type 1 diabetes has increased five-fold over 20 years (Gillespie *et al*., 2004). Furthermore, new research shows that the UK now ranks fifth out of 88 countries in the incidence of type 1 diabetes in children. A league table compiled by the charity Diabetes UK from data from the International Diabetes Federation shows that Finland tops the international league table with a rate of 57.6 per 100,000 children in 2011. Sweden is next with a rate of 43.1, then Saudi Arabia 31.4, and Norway 27.9 and then the UK with 24.5 children in every 100,000 diagnosed (Iacobucci, 2013). Type 1 diabetes is the most common form of the disease in children; over 90 per cent of children under the age of 16 with diabetes have type 1. However, type 2 diabetes (normally affecting adults in the post 40 age group) now seems to be emerging in young adults too at the level of a global epidemic driven by the increasing burden of obesity (Wilmot *et al*., 2010; Song, 2012). This raises the possibility of a serious public health challenge in the next few decades.

Between 1996 and 2011, the number of people diagnosed with diabetes rose from 1.4 to 2.9 million in the UK. An estimated 850,000 people are thought to have the disease but not yet know it. If current trends continue by 2025 it is estimated that five million people in the UK will have diabetes (Diabetes UK, 2012). A report published in the journal *Diabetic Medicine* projects that the NHS's annual spending on diabetes will increase from £9.8 billion to £16.9 billion over the next 25 years, this rise means that **in 2035, the NHS could be spending 17 per cent of its entire budget on treating diabetes** (Hex *et al*., 2012).

The global rise in diabetes is epidemic. In 1985 an estimated 30 million people worldwide had diabetes; a decade later this figure had increased to 135 million and by 2000 an estimated 171 million people had diabetes. In 2011, 347 million people worldwide were affected and the WHO projects that diabetes will be the seventh leading cause of death in 2030 (WHO, 2013b). The increase in diabetes is attributed to a range of factors including population growth, ageing, unhealthy diets that are high in saturated fat and cholesterol, obesity and lack of physical exercise.

Diabetes has become one of the major causes of premature illness and death in many, but not all, countries. Indeed, diabetes occurs much more in some parts of the world, principally in developed countries. Diabetes tends to occur more in cultures consuming diets high in animal fats and less in cultures consuming diets high in complex carbohydrates. As carbohydrate intake increases and saturated animal fat intake decreases from country to country, the number of deaths from type 2 diabetes plummets from 20.4 to 2.9 people per 100,000 (Campbell and Campbell, 2005).

In England and Wales, the rates of diabetes fell markedly between 1940 and 1950. This is because during the Second World War, and in the period following it, people tended to eat less fat and sugar and more plant foods, and therefore more fibre, antioxidants, complex carbohydrates, vitamins and minerals (Trowell, 1974). All available land was used; many people grew their own vegetables and vegetable patches were cultivated all over the country. Gardens, flowerbeds and parks were dug up and planted with vegetables; even the moat around the Tower of London (drained in 1843) was used for growing vegetables. Then as rationing came to an end and people moved away from whole grains towards a more processed diet, rates of diabetes increased again (Trowell, 1974). The conclusion must be that a high-carbohydrate, low-fat plant-based diet offers some protection against type 2 diabetes.

The risk factors for type 2 diabetes (obesity, poor diet and lack of exercise) are well-documented and there are many steps people can take to limit their chances of developing type 2 diabetes. One obvious step is to reduce the amount of saturated fat in the diet, this means cutting down on meat and dairy and increasing the intake of fruit, vegetables, whole grains, pulses, nuts and seeds. Simple lifestyle measures have been shown to be effective in preventing or delaying the onset of type 2 diabetes.

To help prevent type 2 diabetes and its complications, the WHO recommends the following:

- Achieve and maintain healthy body weight
- Be physically active – at least 30 minutes of regular, moderate-intensity activity on most days (more activity is required for weight control)
- Eat a healthy diet of between three and five servings of fruit and vegetables a day and reduce sugar and saturated fats intake
- Avoid tobacco use – smoking increases the risk of cardiovascular diseases

(WHO, 2013b).

Prevention of diabetes is crucial to lowering disease incidence and minimising the public health burden. There is a large body of evidence showing that plant-based diets can lower the risk of diabetes. A study of the relationship between diet and chronic disease in a cohort of 34,192 California Seventh-day Adventists revealed that the vegetarian Adventists were much healthier than their meat-eating counterparts: the meat-eaters were twice as likely as the vegetarians to suffer from diabetes (Fraser, 1999). This study also revealed that obesity increased as meat consumption increased; the difference between vegetarian and non-vegetarian men and women was 6.4kg and 5.5kg respectively (Fraser, 1999). More recently, a meta-analysis of studies examining the role of diet and lifestyle in diabetes prevention found that diets rich in whole-grain, high-fibre cereal products and non-oil-seed pulses (chick peas, beans, peas and lentils) are beneficial, whereas, frequent meat consumption was found to increase the risk (Psaltopoulou et al., 2010). They also found that four cups per day of filtered coffee or tea reduced diabetes risk but that alcoholic beverages should not exceed 1-3 drinks per day. They concluded that obesity is the most important factor accounting for more than half of new diabetes cases; even modest weight loss has a favourable effect in preventing diabetes and physical exercise, with or without diet, contributes to a healthier lifestyle and lowers the risk.

Vegetarian and vegan diets offer significant benefits for diabetes management. One study compared the effects of a low-fat vegan diet with that of a conventional diabetes diet on glycaemia, weight and plasma lipids in a clinical trial (Barnard et al., 2009). Type 2 diabetics were randomly assigned either a low-fat vegan diet or a diet following American Diabetes Association guidelines. Their weight and plasma lipids were measured at the start, middle and end of the 74-week trial. Both groups lost weight but those on the conventional diet had restricted calorie intake whilst the vegan group did not. Both diets were associated with a sustained drop in plasma lipid concentrations. The reduction in triglycerides (fats in blood) in the vegan group was substantial as was the decrease in cholesterol levels (the total cholesterol level fell by 0.53mmol/L and 0.18mmol/L in the vegan and conventional diet groups respectively). Around six in 10 adults in England have cholesterol levels of 5mmol/l or above, you should aim to have a cholesterol level under 4mmol/l (BHF, 2013). So a reduction of 0.5mmol/L could be significant in reducing the risk of heart disease. In an analysis controlling for medication

changes, the low-fat vegan diet was found to improve glycaemia and plasma lipids more than the conventional diabetes diet. In other words, the vegan diet offered significantly more benefits.

A further review of the literature revealed how observational studies show that vegetarians are about half as likely to develop diabetes compared with non-vegetarians. They also describe how in clinical trials in individuals with type 2 diabetes, low-fat vegan diets improve glycaemic control to a greater extent than conventional diabetes diets. This beneficial effect is largely due to weight loss but may also be partly attributable to the reduced intake of saturated fats and high-glycaemic-index foods coupled to the increased intake of dietary fibre and vegetable protein. Vegetarian and vegan diets also improve plasma lipid concentrations and have been shown to reverse atherosclerosis progression, thus lowering the risk of heart disease (Barnard et al., 2009a).

Further studies confirm the beneficial role of plant-based diets in the prevention and treatment of diabetes. A review of both observational studies and intervention trials concluded that a low-fat, plant-based diet can improve control of weight, glycaemia and cardiovascular risk. The authors of this review concluded that vegetarian and vegan diets present potential advantages in managing type 2 diabetes that merit the attention of individuals with diabetes and their caregivers (Trapp and Barnard, 2010). In summary, the current literature indicates that vegetarian and vegan diets present huge potential advantages for the management of type 2 diabetes.

The importance of high-fibre diets in diabetes has been studied extensively since the 1970s by James Anderson, Professor of Medicine at the University of Kentucky. Anderson used a high-fibre, high-carbohydrate low-fat diet to treat 25 type 1 and 25 type 2 diabetics (Anderson, 1986). The experimental diet consisted mostly of whole plant foods (although it did contain a small amount of meat). After three weeks, Anderson measured blood sugar levels, weight and cholesterol levels and calculated their medication requirements. The results were astounding. Remember in type 1 diabetes no insulin is produced so it seems unlikely that a change in diet would help. However, Anderson's patients required 40 per cent less insulin medication than they had needed before the trial. In addition to this, their cholesterol levels dropped by an average of 30 per cent too. This is just as important in lowering the risk factors for secondary outcomes of diabetes such as

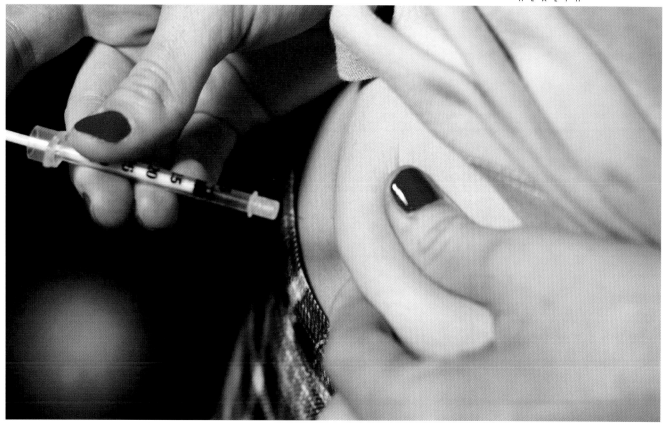

heart disease and stroke. Type 2 diabetes is generally more treatable and the results among the type 2 patients were even more impressive: 24 out of the 25 participants consuming the high-fibre, low-fat diet were able to stop taking their insulin medication completely! These benefits were not of a temporary nature, indeed they were sustained over time in a group of 14 diabetic men continuing on the high-carbohydrate, high-fibre diet for four years (Story *et al.*, 1985).

The evidence is overwhelming: a high-carbohydrate, high-fibre diet provides effective, positive and safe treatment for diabetes and lowers the associated risk for coronary artery disease (Anderson *et al.*, 1990). More recent studies have shown increasing dietary fibre in the diet of patients with type 2 diabetes is beneficial and should be encouraged as a disease management strategy (Anderson *et al.*, 2004; Barnard *et al.*, 2009; Post *et al.*, 2012). Of course it should be noted that this is not a special diet for diabetics; most people would benefit from increasing their fibre intake while reducing the amount of dietary fat they consume.

As stated, it is thought that type 1 diabetes involves a genetic susceptibility coupled to an environmental trigger. It has been suggested that an increased environmental pressure may reduce the need for a strong genetic susceptibility in order for type 1 diabetes to develop (Vehik *et al.*, 2008). Modern molecular genetics has enabled scientists to identify genes linked to type 1 diabetes and develop a hierarchy of susceptibility based on the number of these genes that a person carries. People carrying a

high proportion of the high risk genes are referred to as having a 'high-risk HLA genotype'. Researchers from the Diabetes and Metabolism Division of Medicine at the University of Bristol looked at the frequency of these high risk genes in a group of 194 patients who were diagnosed with type 1 diabetes as children over 50 years ago (between 1922 and 1946). They compared them to a group of 582 age-matched and sex-matched individuals diagnosed between 1985 and 2002. Results showed that the frequency of the high-risk genotype was 12 per cent lower in the individuals diagnosed recently compared with the older group (Gillespie *et al.*, 2004). Other studies from Finland and the US have found a similar disparity (Hermann *et al.*, 2003; Vehik *et al.*, 2008).

So, what does this all mean? The important point here is that increasing environmental exposure is now able to trigger type 1 diabetes in people who are less genetically susceptible than the generation above them. In other words, the rapid rise of type 1 diabetes must be due to a major environmental factor rather than genes.

But what is this elusive environmental trigger? A growing body of evidence suggests it may be a component of the diet. In 2000 an extensive study of children from 40 different countries confirmed a link between diet and incidence of type 1 diabetes (Muntoni *et al.*, 2000). The study set out to examine the relationship between dietary energy from major food groups and incidence of type 1 diabetes. The total energy intake was not associated with type 1 diabetes incidence. However, energy from animal sources (meat and dairy foods) was associated and energy from plant sources was inversely associated with diabetes. This means that the more meat and milk in the diet, the higher the incidence of diabetes and the more plant-based food in the diet, the lower the incidence.

As stated, type 1 diabetes is thought to involve both a genetic predisposition and an environmental trigger. The trigger may be a virus or some component of food. In the early 1990s a Canadian research group suggested that cow's milk proteins might be an important environmental trigger providing specific peptides that share antigenic epitopes with host cell proteins (Martin et al., 1991). This means that the proteins in cow's milk look the same as proteins in our own bodies; these similarities can confuse our immune system and initiate an inappropriate (autoimmune) response that can lead to diabetes.

The milk protein casein is similar in shape to the insulin-producing cells in the pancreas. Because the body may perceive casein as a foreign invader and attack it, it may also start to attack the pancreas cells having confused them for casein, again leading to diabetes (Cavallo et al., 1996). Some studies have suggested that bovine serum albumin (BSA) is the milk protein responsible. In a study of 142 children with type 1 diabetes, all the diabetic patients had higher serum concentrations of anti-BSA antibodies compared to 79 healthy children (Karjalainen et al., 1992). These antibodies may react with proteins on the surface of the beta cells of the pancreas and so interfere with insulin production.

Other studies suggest it is the cow's insulin present in formula milk that increases the risk of type 1 diabetes in infants (Vaarala et al., 1999). Research shows that some infants may be more vulnerable to type 1 diabetes later in life if exposed to cow's milk formula while very young. A Finnish study of children (with at least one close relative with type 1 diabetes) examined whether early exposure to insulin in cow's milk formula increased the risk of type 1 diabetes. Results showed that infants given cow's milk formula at three-months-old had immune systems which reacted far more strongly to cow's insulin (Paronen et al., 2000). This raises concerns that exposure to cow's insulin plays a role in the autoimmune process leading to type 1 diabetes.

A review of the clinical evidence suggests that the incidence of type 1 diabetes is related to the early consumption of cow's milk; children with type 1

diabetes are more likely to have been breastfed for less than three months and to have been exposed to cow's milk protein before four months of age (Gerstein et al., 1994). The avoidance of cow's milk during the first few months of life may reduce the risk of type 1 diabetes. Infants who cannot breastfeed from their mothers may benefit more from taking a plant-based formula such as soya-based formula rather than one based on cow's milk. Other studies support the finding that both early and adolescent exposure to cow's milk may be a trigger for type 1 diabetes (Kimpimaki et al., 2001; Thorsdottir and Ramel, 2003).

Further evidence suggesting that the early exposure to cow's milk in infancy (including cow's milk infant formula) may be a trigger for type 1 diabetes in some children was provided in a substantial review of 27 case-control studies and one prospective cohort study looking at the associations of breastfeeding and/or the early introduction of cow's milk and formula with the development of type 1 diabetes. Eight of the studies showed that breastfeeding can protect against type 1 diabetes while seven additional studies emphasised that a short period or absence of breastfeeding could be a risk factor for type 1 diabetes. The authors concluded that a short duration and/or a lack of breastfeeding may constitute a risk factor for the development of type 1 diabetes later in life (Patelarou et al., 2012).

The hunt for the elusive environmental trigger responsible for the global rise in the incidence of type 1 diabetes continues. Theories include: the hygiene hypothesis (a lack of early childhood exposure to infectious agents and parasites weakens immunity and increases susceptibility to allergic and autoimmune diseases), a viral agent, vitamin D deficiency and the breast milk versus cow's milk argument. It may be that no single factor is responsible for the increase in the incidence of diabetes all over the world, a multi-factorial process might be involved and there may be some overlap between the various hypotheses (Ergo, 2013). However, taken together, the evidence suggests that avoiding milk and milk products may offer protection from diabetes (types 1 and 2).

For more information see Viva!Health's fully-referenced scientific report *The Big-D: Defeating Diabetes through Diet* and easy-to-read guide *The Big-D: defeating diabetes with the D-Diet* at www.vegetarian.org.uk/campaigns/diabetes.

Dementia

Obesity is epidemic in Western societies and constitutes a major public health concern. A study published in the *British Journal of Medicine* reports that being obese during middle-age can increase the risk of developing dementia later in life (Whitmer *et al.*, 2005). The research is based on data collected from detailed health checks made on 10,276 men and women between 1964 and 1973 (when they were aged 40 to 45). Dementia was diagnosed in seven per cent of participants between 1994 and 2003. Results showed that being obese increased the risk of dementia by a whopping 74 per cent while being overweight increased it by 35 per cent. The link between obesity and dementia in women was stronger than that in men.

This is in agreement with a Swedish study which found that the higher a woman's body mass index (BMI), the greater the risk of dementia (Gustafson *et al.*, 2003). In this study the relationship between BMI and dementia risk was investigated in 392 Swedish adults who were assessed between the ages of 70 and 88. During the 18-year study, 93 participants were diagnosed as having dementia. Women who developed dementia had a higher average BMI compared to women without dementia. For every one unit increase in BMI at age 70 years, the risk of dementia increased by 36 per cent.

A substantial body of evidence now shows that obesity is a risk factor for dementia. However, it has been argued that current forecasts of dementia fail to take the rising obesity levels into account. A review of studies on the association between midlife obesity and dementia found that, compared to normal weight, being overweight or obese in midlife, increases the risk of dementia later in life by 34 and 91 per cent respectively. It was predicted that dementia levels in the US and China would be nine and 19 per cent higher respectively than previously forecast (Loef *et al.*, 2013). The authors of this review conclude that the increase in midlife obesity levels will contribute significantly to the future prevalence of dementia and suggest that public health measures to reduce midlife obesity should be regarded as also being primary prevention measures to reduce the risk of dementia. This raises very real concerns that the current obesity epidemic could lead to a steep rise in the numbers of people suffering from dementia in the future. The evidence suggests that eating a healthy plant-based diet and leading a healthy lifestyle could help to reduce the risk of dementia (See Overweight and obesity).

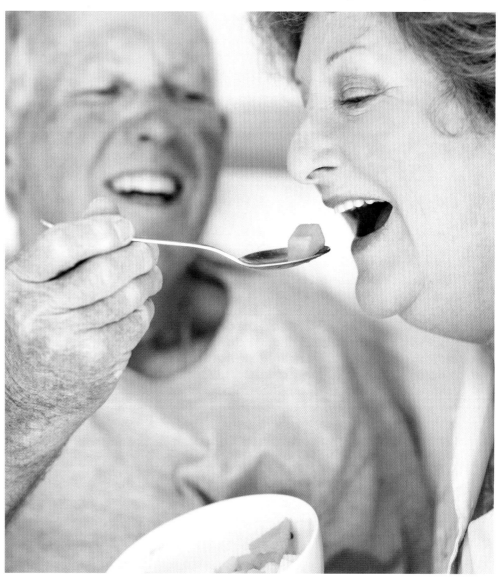

Ear Infection

The most common type of ear infection (*otitis media*) affects the middle ear, the space between the eardrum and the inner ear. The middle ear is usually filled with air but it can fill up with fluid (during a cold for example) and ear infections happen when bacteria, viruses or fungi infect the fluid and cause swelling in the ear. Ear infections are common in childhood and can be extremely painful causing a considerable amount of distress. Chronic *otitis media* is when ear infections keep recurring, for example glue ear is a type of chronic otitis media. *Otitis media* usually reoccurs several times during childhood years. One third of children will have six or more episodes of *otitis media* by the time they are seven years old. The condition occurs less often as the child gets older. It would be unusual for children over the age of seven to be affected by further episodes (NHS Choices, 2012m). Complications of middle ear infection are now less common than they were in the past. However, it can be a serious problem; otitis media with effusion (glue ear) is the most common cause of hearing impairment in childhood (NICE, 2011). Symptoms vary with time and age, hearing loss usually resolves over several weeks or months, but may be more persistent if in both ears, may lead to educational, language and behavioural problems.

Ear infections are often linked to colds or other problems of the respiratory system. However, some reports link ear infections to food allergies (Hurst, 1998; Aydogan *et al.*, 2004; Doner *et al.*, 2004). Researchers from Georgetown University in the US examined the role of food allergy in ear infection in 104 children with recurrent ear problems (Nsouli *et al.*, 1994). The children were tested for food allergies and those who tested positive excluded that particular food for 16 weeks, then reintroduced it. Results showed that 78 per cent of the children with ear problems also had food allergies, the most common allergenic foods were cow's milk (38 per cent), wheat (33 per cent), egg white (25 per cent), peanut (20 per cent) and soya (17 per cent). 86 per cent of these children responded well to eliminating the offending food, and of these, 94 per cent suffered a recurrence of ear problems on reintroducing the offending food.

A different approach was taken in a Finnish study of 56 children with cow's milk allergy and 204 children without cow's milk allergy. These researchers examined the occurrence of ear infection in children known to have cow's milk allergy. Results showed that 27 per cent of those with the allergy suffered from recurrent ear infections compared to just 12 per cent of those who did not have the allergy (Juntti *et al.*, 1999). It was concluded that children with cow's milk allergy experience significantly more ear infections.

Dr John James of the Colorado Allergy and Asthma Centres in the US suggests that food allergies can cause inflammation in the nasal passages and lead to the build-up of fluid in the middle ear, but he acknowledges that the link between food allergy and ear infection may be hard to prove (James, 2004). A recent review stated how a large body of epidemiologic evidence now supports a role for allergic rhinitis (allergic inflammation of the nasal airways) as a possible cause of *otitis media*. Evidence also supports a role for histamine (a compound that triggers the inflammatory response) in both conditions (Skoner *et al.*, 2009). The authors of this study say that given the strong likelihood of allergy as a risk factor for *otitis media*, allergic rhinitis patients should be evaluated for *otitis media* and vice versa.

In 2009 the American Dietetic Association reported that for infants, breastfeeding is associated with a reduced risk of otitis media (along with a reduced risk of gastroenteritis, respiratory illness, sudden infant death syndrome, necrotising enterocolitis, obesity and hypertension. They say that exclusive breastfeeding provides optimal nutrition and health protection for the first six months of life and breastfeeding with complementary foods from six months until at least 12 months of age is the ideal feeding pattern for infants (James *et al.*, 2009). More studies are needed to examine the relationship between food allergy and ear infection but the possibility of cow's milk allergy should be considered in all cases of ear infection, particularly in children.

Food Poisoning

Food poisoning is a common, often mild, but sometimes deadly illness. It is caused by the consumption of food or drink that is contaminated with bacteria, parasites or viruses. Most cases result from bacterial contamination. Food poisoning happens in one of two ways: either in the food (for example in undercooked meat or unpasteurised milk), or on the food (if it is prepared by someone who has not washed their hands). The length of the incubation period (the time between swallowing the bacteria and symptoms appearing) varies from hours to days, depending on the type of bacteria and how many were swallowed. The most common symptoms of food poisoning are sickness, vomiting, abdominal pain and diarrhoea. It's difficult to know exactly how many people get food poisoning because mild cases often go unreported but the Food Standards Agency estimates that food poisoning affects up to 5.5 million people in the UK each year (NHS Choices, 2013f). It usually lasts for less than three days, but can continue for up to a week. The greatest danger lies in the loss of fluids and salts from prolonged diarrhoea. The results can be deadly in infants and over 60s. Also, in these patients, the bacteria may enter the bloodstream infecting other parts of the body and may cause death unless the person is treated promptly with antibiotics.

Some toxins can cause food poisoning within a much shorter time than described above. In these cases, vomiting is the main symptom. Foods particularly susceptible to contamination if not handled, stored or cooked properly include:

- Raw meat and poultry
- Raw eggs
- Raw shellfish
- Unpasteurised milk
- 'Ready to eat' foods, such as cooked sliced meats, pâté, soft cheeses and pre-packed sandwiches

Source: NHS Choices, 2013e.

Most cases of food poisoning are related to the consumption of animal products (meat, poultry, eggs, fish and dairy) as plants tend not to harbour the types of bacteria capable of causing food poisoning in humans. Intensive animal husbandry technologies, introduced to minimise production costs, have led to the emergence of new zoonotic diseases; animal diseases that can be transmitted to humans (WHO, 2013c). *Escherichia coli* (*E. coli*) O157 was identified for the first time in 1979 and has since

caused illness and deaths (especially among children) owing to its presence (in several countries) in minced beef, unpasteurised cider, cow's milk, manure-contaminated lettuce and alfalfa and manure-contaminated drinking-water (WHO, 2013c). The potential sources of *E. coli* contamination of fruit (cider apples) are numerous. One possible source may be bird droppings; birds have been shown to spread various food-borne pathogens including *Campylobacter*, *Salmonella*, *Vibrio cholerae* and *Listeria* species. Another possibility is windfall apples being exposed to animal faeces. The contamination of damaged apples with *E. coli* O157:H7 can also be spread by fruit flies and then fruit-to-fruit transmission by fruit flies ensures the infection spreads (Janisiewicz *et al.*, 1999). Indeed research shows that flies can transmit foodborne pathogens and that the areas of higher risk are those in closer proximity to animal production sites (Barreiro *et al.*, 2013). In a joint report between the FSA Scotland and the Scottish Executive it was noted that the main source of *E. coli* O157 is from cattle and sheep, but that more cases of *E. coli* O157 are now associated with environmental contamination, including contact with animal faeces or contamination by faeces of water supplies, than with food (FSA/SE, 2001). If plants do cause food poisoning it is generally because they have been contaminated with animal excreta, human sewerage or handled with dirty hands during preparation. Safe disposal of manure from large-scale animal and poultry production facilities is a growing food safety problem in much of the world (WHO, 2013c).

Food can become contaminated at any stage during production, processing or cooking, for example, food poisoning can be caused by:

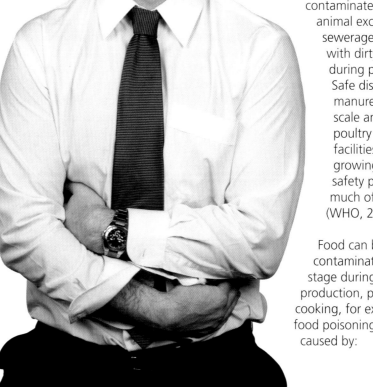

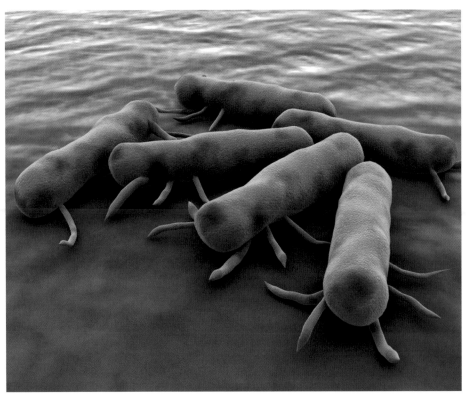

- Not cooking food thoroughly (particularly poultry, pork, burgers, sausages and kebabs)
- Not storing food that needs to be chilled at below 5°C correctly
- Leaving cooked food for too long at warm temperatures
- Someone who is ill or who has dirty hands touching the food
- Eating food that has passed its 'use by' date
- Cross-contamination (the spread of bacteria, such as *E.coli*, from contaminated foods)

Source: NHS Choices, 2013e.

The most common cause of food poisoning in the UK is the bacterium *Campylobacter*, which are usually found on raw or undercooked meat (particularly poultry), unpasteurised milk and untreated water. Undercooked chicken liver and liver pâté are also common sources. The next most common cause is *Salmonella*, which are often found in raw meat and poultry, they can also be passed into eggs and unpasteurised milk. *Listeria* bacteria may be found in a range of chilled, ready-to-eat food, including: pre-packed sandwiches, pâté, butter, soft cheeses (such as brie, camembert or others with a similar rind), soft blue cheese, cooked sliced meats and smoked salmon. *E. coli* are found in the digestive systems of many animals, including humans. Most strains are harmless but some strains can cause serious illness. Most cases of *E. coli* food poisoning occur after eating undercooked beef (particularly mince, burgers and meatballs) or drinking unpasteurised milk (NHS Choices, 2013f).

The virus most commonly linked to gastrointestinal illness is the norovirus (also known as the vomiting bug). It is easily transmitted from person to person, from contaminated food or water. Raw shellfish, particularly oysters can be a source of viral contamination. A study funded by the Foods Standards Agency found that three-quarters of oysters sampled from harvesting beds within UK waters contained norovirus (albeit at low levels in half the samples). The FSA advises that older people, pregnant women, very young children and people who are unwell should avoid eating raw or lightly cooked shellfish to reduce their risk of food poisoning (NHS Choices, 2013f).

In the Food Standards Agency's Annual Report to the Chief Scientist 2012-2013, it was reported that of the five major pathogens monitored by the Agency (campylobacter, *Listeria monocytogenes*, norovirus, *E. coli* O157 and salmonella), campylobacter remains the most frequently reported cause of foodborne disease accounting for 60 per cent of reported cases in England and Wales and the highest proportion of hospitalisations (92 per cent). Although foodborne illness due to *Listeria monocytogenes* is relatively rare (less than one per cent), it is associated with the highest mortality at 30 per cent (FSA, 2013a).

The Food Standards Agency's current best estimate suggests that there are around one million cases of foodborne illness in the UK each year, resulting in 20,000 hospital admissions and contributing to around 500 deaths. However, many illnesses go unreported and their report states that around 25 per cent of the population suffer from an episode of intestinal infectious disease each year; equivalent to 17 million cases annually. The public health impact of gastrointestinal infection continues to be significant; the estimated cost for England and Wales in 2011 was £1.6 billion (FSA, 2013a).

Listeria is an opportunistic pathogen that can cause severe illness (listeriosis) in vulnerable groups such as pregnant women, babies, the elderly and people with reduced immunity. The Government advises pregnant women to avoid soft mould-ripened cheese, such as Camembert and Brie, blue cheese and all types of meat pâté. Other bacteria that can cause food poisoning include species of *Staphylococcus* and *Clostridium*. Certain strains of otherwise normal

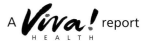

intestinal bacteria can cause food poisoning. For example, *E. coli* is usually harmless but the strain *E. coli* O157 can cause kidney failure and death.

The majority of food poisoning cases in the UK are caused by consuming contaminated meat or dairy products. For example, of the *Staphylococcal* food poisonings reported in the UK between 1969 and 1990, 53 per cent were due to meat products (especially ham), 22 per cent were due to poultry, eight per cent were due to milk products, seven per cent to fish and shellfish and 3.5 per cent to eggs (Wieneke *et al.*, 1993). While most cases of food poisoning are associated with meat and poultry, the link between milk products and food poisoning should not be discounted: 20 separate outbreaks of food poisoning in England and Wales associated with the consumption of milk and dairy products were reported to the Public Health Laboratory Service Communicable Disease Surveillance Centre between 1992 and 1996 (Djuretic *et al.*, 1997). 600 people were affected and over 45 were admitted to hospital. *Salmonella* species were responsible for 11 of the outbreaks, *Campylobacter* species for five, *E. coli* O157 for three and *Cryptosporidium parvum* for one. Outbreaks were associated with hotels, a psychogeriatric hospital, schools, a Royal Air Force base, a farm visit, an outdoor festival and milk supplied directly from farms. Milk was implicated in 16 of the outbreaks, 10 of which were associated with unpasteurised milk. Two outbreaks were associated with eating contaminated ice-cream and two with eating contaminated cheese.

In 2010, it was reported that since 2001, an increase in the number of listeriosis cases has been observed in several EU countries, including England and Wales, predominantly in the over-60s population (Little *et al.*, 2010). The main culprits for the overall population and over 60's were given as follows: mixed sandwiches and pre-packed salads (23.1 and 22 per cent respectively); finfish (16.8 and 14.7 per cent) and beef (15.3 and 11.2 per cent). For pregnancy-associated cases, beef (12.3 per cent), milk and milk products (11.8 per cent), and finfish (11.2 per cent) were more important sources of infection. Food poisoning may result from milk and milk products if they have not been properly heated (pasteurised) or if they have become contaminated following pasteurisation. A report published in the *New England Journal of Medicine* reported how 142 cases of listeriosis in Los Angeles in 1985 led to 48 deaths (Linnan, 1988). An extensive investigation traced the source to a cheese factory where it was

found that a Mexican-style soft cheese had been contaminated with unpasteurised milk.

Bacteria are too small to see and they do not taste or smell of anything so it is difficult to detect their presence. The risk of food poisoning can be minimised by following some basic hygiene rules. This means washing hands before handling food, washing salads thoroughly (to remove contaminating bacteria from manure for example), making sure all food is covered and chilled. If meat is to be consumed it must be thawed and cooked properly to kill harmful bacteria. It is important to keep raw meat (and its juices) away from other foods.

The Centers for Disease Control and Prevention (CDC) in Atlanta, US is a national public health institute that focuses on disease control and prevention. The CDC state that raw (unpasteurised) milk can carry harmful bacteria and other germs and that while it is possible to get foodborne illnesses from many different foods, they say that raw milk is one of the riskiest of all. Bacteria such as *E. coli*, *Campylobacter* and *Salmonella* can contaminate milk from cows, sheep and goats. Animals that carry these germs usually appear healthy. Getting sick from raw milk can mean many days of diarrhoea, stomach cramping, and vomiting. Less commonly, it can mean kidney failure, paralysis, chronic disorders and even death. A person can develop severe or even life-threatening diseases, such as Guillain-Barré syndrome, which can cause paralysis and haemolytic uremic syndrome, which can result in kidney failure and stroke (CDC, 2013).

Milk contamination may occur from:

- Cow faeces coming into direct contact with the milk
- Infection of the cow's udder (mastitis)
- Cow diseases (eg bovine tuberculosis)
- Bacteria that live on the skin of cows
- Environmental contamination (eg faeces, dirt, processing equipment)
- Insects, rodents and other animal vectors
- Humans (eg by cross-contamination from soiled clothing or boots)

Source: CDC, 2013.

Good hygienic practices during milking may reduce, but not eliminate, the risk of milk contamination. However, as the CDC state, dairy farms are a reservoir for illness-causing bacteria. No matter what precautions farmers take and even if their raw milk tests come back negative, they cannot guarantee that the milk, or the products made from their milk, are free of harmful germs (CDC, 2013).

Distribution of raw milk is illegal in Scotland. In England it is illegal to sell it from shops or supermarkets but a number of registered producers can sell raw or 'green top' milk, directly to consumers, either from a farm or at a farmers' market or through a delivery service. The number of registered raw cow's drinking milk producers in England and Wales fell from around 570 in 1997 to 102 in 2009 (FSA, 2009). They must display the warning "this product has not been heat-treated and may contain organisms harmful to health" and the dairy must conform to higher hygiene standards than dairies producing only pasteurised milk. Avoiding unpasteurised milk, raw eggs and undercooked meat further reduces the risk of food poisoning. Of course the safest option is to follow a plant-based diet free of red meat, poultry, fish, milk and eggs. Excluding animal foods from the diet will dramatically decrease the risk of food poisoning.

Gallstones

Gallstones are solid pieces of stone-like material usually made of cholesterol that form in the gall bladder, which is a small organ on the right hand side of the body, below the liver. It stores a green liquid called bile, which is produced by the liver to help the body digest fats. As we eat, bile is released from the gall bladder into the intestines through a thin tube called the bile duct. Gallstones are formed when some of the chemicals stored in the gall bladder harden into a solid mass. They may be as small as a grain of sand or as large as a golf ball. Some people may have one large stone while others may have many small ones. Gallstones are the most common cause of emergency hospital admission for people with abdominal pain. About eight per cent of the adult population has gallstones and 50,000 people a year have an operation to remove their gallbladder (NHS Choices, 2012o).

Gallstones are made up from a mixture of water, cholesterol and other fats, bile salts and the pigment bilirubin. They occur when the composition of the bile is abnormal, the outlet from the gall bladder is blocked (perhaps by infection), or if there is a family history of gallstones. Gallstones can cause inflammation of the gall bladder (cholecystitis), which may then block the bile duct leading to obstructive jaundice. The passage of a gallstone

along the bile duct to the duodenum can be extremely painful.

Obesity is a major risk factor for gallstones, especially in women, who are two to three times as likely as men to develop gallstones. Risk also increases with age; people over 40 are at a higher risk. Diet is also a causal factor. A study published in the British Medical Journal in 1985 reported that meat-eaters are twice as likely to develop gallstones as vegetarians (Pixley et al., 1985). Since then the low incidence of gallstones in vegetarians compared to meat-eaters has been reported (Key et al., 1999). Indeed vegetarian diets have been shown to be beneficial for both the prevention and treatment of gallstones (Leitzmann, 2005). The main risk factors appear to be low fibre intake, high saturated fat and cholesterol intake and obesity. An Australian study reported an inverse association between dietary fibre and gallstones (Segasothy and Phillips, 2000). In other words, the more fibre in the diet, the lower the risk of gallstones. Polish researchers examined the diets of patients suffering from gallstones and found that they were characterised by their low fibre diet (Ostrowska et al., 2005). Patients with gallstones ate less wholemeal products, fruit and vegetables and pulses. Furthermore, obese women with gallstones ate significantly more milk, yogurt, meat and meat products.

Due to the role that cholesterol appears to play in the formation of gallstones, the UK government recommends that the following fatty foods with high cholesterol content are avoided: meat pies, sausages and fatty cuts of meat, butter and lard, and cakes and biscuits. They recommend a low-fat, high-fibre diet including plenty of fresh fruit and vegetables (at least five portions a day) and wholegrain foods (NHS Choices, 2012p). They also say that there is evidence that regularly eating nuts (such as peanuts or cashews), can help reduce the risk of developing gallstones. Cutting down your drinking to no more than 3-4 units a day for men and 2-3 units a day for women may also reduce the risk.

Insulin-like growth factor 1 (IGF-1)

Insulin-like growth factor 1 (IGF-1) is a hormone produced in the liver and body tissues of mammals. One important role for IGF-1 is to promote cell growth and division, this is important for normal growth and

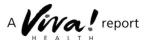
development. It plays an important role in childhood growth and continues to have anabolic effects (the building up of organs and tissues) in adults.

IGF-1 from cows is identical to human IGF-1 in that the amino acid sequence of both molecules is the same (Honegger and Humbel, 1986). Amino acids are the building blocks of proteins and there are 20 different amino acids. All proteins consist of amino acids joined together like beads on a string and the nature of the protein (how it behaves) is determined by the order in which the amino acids occur along the string. In both human and bovine IGF-1 the same 70 amino acids occur in exactly the same order, which may or may not have a significant impact on human health (see below). As previously stated, the use of recombinant bovine somatotrophin (rBST) in cows increases levels of IGF-1 in their milk, however, it should be noted that cow's milk from cows that are not treated with rBST also contains IGF-1. Again, the significance of this is discussed below.

It has been suggested that IGF-1 is not destroyed during pasteurisation. Furthermore it has also been suggested that it is not completely broken down in the gut and that it may cross the intestinal wall in the same way that another hormone, epidermal growth factor (EGF), has been shown to do. EGF is protected from being broken down when food proteins (such as the milk protein casein) block the active sites of the digestive enzymes (Playford *et al*., 1993). This allows the molecule to stay intact and cross the intestinal wall and enter the blood. This raises a theoretical concern that IGF-1 from cow's milk could increase normal blood IGF-1 levels and so increase the risk of certain cancers linked to IGF-1.

However, Professor Jeffrey Holly, Professor of Clinical Sciences at the University of

Bristol says that although bovine IGF-1 is identical to human IGF-1 and in theory some of the IGF-1 that is present in ingested milk may be absorbed un-degraded, it is implausible that this would affect the systemic levels of IGF-1 in humans. Holly states that the dynamics of the IGF-1 system (with a huge circulating reservoir and a large flux primarily due to production from the liver) means that even assuming the extreme estimates of what could be absorbed and not metabolised it would still require consumption of something like 60 litres of milk a day to increase serum levels by the least amount that could be measurable. However, he goes on to say that there are many small peptides and amino acids that are present in milk that potently stimulate hepatic IGF-1 expression and pituitary growth hormone release (Holly, 2013). In other words, drinking milk increases IGF-1 production from the liver which in turn leads to an increase in the levels present in the blood.

Milk is designed as the only food between birth and weaning and is designed to sustain the rapid growth that occurs at this stage of life. Holly states that his studies and those of others have consistently found that, of all the components of human diet, milk and dairy products have the greatest effects on IGF-1 levels. So it is not the presence of IGF-1 in milk that matters but rather the impact of milk on stimulating human IGF-1 production within individuals who consume milk and dairy products. He also points out that there is similar confusion over dairy cows treated with rBST (in the US), the milk from such cows has higher levels of bovine growth hormone and bovine IGF-1 but neither are likely to alter the effects on humans consuming such milk.

Whether cow's milk ingestion increases IGF-1 levels in humans by bovine IGF-1 crossing the gut wall, or (as seems more likely) other components in milk initiating a rapid rise in human IGF-1 production from the liver, the net effect is the same; if you drink cow's milk, you end up with higher levels of IGF-1 in your blood (see below).

As stated, IGF-1 regulates cell growth, development and division; it can stimulate growth in both normal and cancerous cells. Even small increases in serum levels of IGF-1 in humans are associated with increased risk for several common cancers including cancers of the breast, prostate, lung and colon (Wu et al., 2002). The link between IGF-1 and cancer is becoming increasingly apparent in the scientific literature.

In the first prospective study to investigate the relationship between the risk of breast cancer and circulating IGF-1 levels, researchers at Harvard Medical School analysed blood samples originally collected from 32,826 women aged between 43 and 69 years during 1989 and 1990. From this group, 397 women were later diagnosed with breast cancer. Analysis of IGF-1 levels in samples collected from these women compared to samples from 620 controls (without breast cancer) revealed a positive relationship between circulating IGF-1 levels and the risk of breast cancer among premenopausal (but not postmenopausal) women. It was concluded that plasma IGF-1 concentrations may be useful in the identification of premenopausal women at high risk of breast cancer (Hankinson et al., 1998a).

To investigate the link between prostate cancer risk and plasma IGF-1 levels, a study was conducted on 152 men with prostate cancer and 152 men without the disease. Analysis revealed a strong positive association between IGF-1 levels and prostate cancer risk (Chan et al., 1998). In agreement, a Swedish study compared IGF-1 levels in 210 prostate cancer patients with those in 224 men without the disease and found that there was a strong positive correlation between the risk of prostate cancer and raised serum levels of IGF-1. It was concluded that high levels of IGF-1 may be an important predictor for risk of prostate cancer (Wolk et al., 1998).

In a study into the link between the risk of lung cancer and IGF-1, serum IGF-1 levels were measured in 204 lung cancer patients registered at the University of Texas M.D. Anderson Cancer Centre and compared to those in 218 people without lung cancer. Results showed that high levels of IGF-1 were associated with an increased risk of lung cancer (Yu et al., 1999).

In order to assess colorectal cancer risk in relation to IGF-1, a research group at Harvard Medical School analysed blood plasma samples originally collected from a pool of 14,916 men. In a 14-year follow-up of these men, 193 had been diagnosed with colorectal cancer. Analysis of IGF-1 levels in samples taken from these men and 318 controls revealed an increased risk for colorectal cancer among the men who had the highest levels of circulating IGF-1 and it was concluded that circulating IGF-1 is related to future risk of colorectal cancer (Ma et al., 1999).

In summary, the literature strongly supports a link between high circulating IGF-1 levels and cancer, but what has this to do with the consumption of cow's milk and dairy products? The answer is a lot: circulating IGF-1 levels are higher in people who consume milk and dairy products. Researchers at Bristol University investigating the association of diet with IGF-1 in 344 disease-free men found that raised levels of IGF-1 were associated with higher intakes of milk, dairy products and calcium while lower levels of IGF-1 were associated with high vegetable consumption, particularly tomatoes. In their study, published in the British Journal of Cancer, it was concluded that IGF-1 may mediate some diet-cancer associations (Gunnell et al., 2003).

US researchers from Harvard Medical School and Bringham and Women's Hospital in Boston also investigated the link between IGF-1 levels and diet. They examined circulating IGF-1 levels in 1,037 healthy women. The most consistent finding was a positive association between circulating IGF-1 and protein intake; this was largely attributable to cow's milk intake (Holmes et al., 2002). In another study, researchers at the Fred Hutchinson Cancer Research Centre in Washington investigated the link between plasma levels of IGF-1 and lifestyle factors in 333 people thought to be representative of the general population. They too found that milk consumption was linked to IGF-1 levels (Morimoto et al., 2005). One study actually quantified the effect of cow's milk on circulating IGF-1 levels in 54 Danish boys aged 2.5 years. In this study an increase in cow's milk intake from 200 to 600ml per day corresponded to a massive 30 per cent increase in circulating IGF-1. In agreement with Holly's research, it was concluded that milk contains certain compounds that stimulate IGF-1 concentrations (Hoppe et al., 2004). An even earlier study concurred that cow's milk contains many bioactive compounds such as hormones and cytokines, growth factors, and many bioactive peptides (Playford et al., 2000), which may also affect IGF-1 levels.

In conclusion, the research shows that nutrition has an important role in determining serum IGF-1 levels (Yaker et al., 2005). Whether the increase in IGF-1

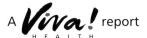

caused by cow's milk occurs directly (by IGF-1 crossing the gut wall), or indirectly (as a result of the action of other factors), the research is clear. The consumption of cow's milk and milk products is linked to increased levels of IGF-1, which in turn are linked to various cancers. In time, the molecular mechanisms underlying these links will inevitably be teased out.

Kidney Disease

The kidneys are two bean-shaped organs located in the lower back. Kidneys filter the blood to remove unwanted waste products broken down from our food and drink. They also remove excess liquid to help maintain correct fluid balance in the body.

There are many diseases and conditions that can affect the kidney function: kidney inflammation (glomerulonephritis); kidney infection (such as pyelonephritis); genetic disorders (such as polycystic kidney disease); hardening of the kidney due to a disease of the arteries (nephrosclerosis); kidney failure due to atherosclerosis (plaques forming in the arteries supplying the kidneys); autoimmune diseases (such as systemic lupus erythematosus); malaria; yellow fever; certain medicines; mechanical blockages (kidney stones) and physical injury.

Surveys have revealed that mild forms of kidney disease are surprisingly common among the general population. The global epidemic of type 2 diabetes has led to an alarming increase in the number of people with chronic kidney disease. The prevalence of chronic kidney disease is estimated to be eight to 16 per cent worldwide (Jha *et al.*, 2013). There may be no apparent symptoms, although small amounts of blood or protein may pass through the damaged filters in the kidneys into the urine. Such small amounts of blood and protein in the urine are not visible but can be detected by certain medical tests.

Normally protein is filtered out by the kidneys and no protein is excreted into the urine. However, when the kidneys are damaged, protein may pass into the urine. Other symptoms include retention of water in the body, called nephrotic syndrome. In some cases the damage to the kidney can be so severe that it leads to a build-up of waste in the body and ultimately kidney failure. The symptoms of kidney failure include tiredness, sickness and vomiting.

Certain kidney disorders can lead to the formation of a kidney stone (renal calculi), a small hard mass in the kidney that forms from mineral deposits in the urine. Stones may form when there is a high level of calcium, oxalate or uric acid in the urine; a lack of citrate in the urine; or insufficient water in the kidneys to dissolve waste products.

Traditionally, a low-calcium diet has been recommended to reduce the strain on the kidneys in kidney stone patients. However, over time a low-calcium diet can cause problems in terms of bone health. In the last decade, attention has switched to the effects of animal protein on kidney stone formation. Several studies now suggest that a diet characterised by normal-calcium, low-animal protein and low-salt levels is more effective than the traditional low-calcium diet for the prevention of kidney stones in some people.

The relationship between an animal protein-rich diet and kidney stone formation was investigated by researchers at the Centre in Mineral Metabolism and Clinical Research at the Department of Internal Medicine in Dallas, Texas (Breslau, 1988). In this study, 15 young healthy participants were studied for three 12-day dietary periods during which their diet contained vegetable protein, vegetable and egg protein, or animal protein. While all three diets were constant with respect to sodium, potassium, calcium, phosphorus, magnesium and the total quantity of protein, they had progressively higher sulphur contents (due to the increased sulphur content of animal proteins compared to that of plant proteins). As the sulphur content of the diet increased, urinary calcium excretion increased from 103mg per day on the vegetarian diet to 150mg per day on the animal protein diet. The animal protein-rich diet was associated with the highest excretion of uric acid and therefore conferred an increased risk for uric acid stones (but not for calcium oxalate stones). The link between animal protein and kidney stone formation has since been demonstrated in both men (Curhan *et al.*, 1993; Taylor *et al.*, 2004) and women (Curhan *et al.*, 1997).

More recently, the Researchers from Harvard Medical School prospectively examined the relationship between a Dietary Approaches to Stop Hypertension (DASH) style diet and the incident of kidney stones in three large cohorts: The Health Professionals Follow-up Study (45,821 men with 18 years of follow-up), The Nurses' Health Study I (94,108 older women and 18 years of follow-up), and The Nurses' Health Study II (101,837 younger women with 14 years of follow-up). The DASH diet is high in fruits and vegetables, moderate in low-fat dairy products and low in animal protein (but with a substantial amount of plant protein from pulses and nuts). Over a combined 50 years of follow-up, they documented 5,645 kidney stones in the three cohorts. Results showed that the consumption of a DASH-style diet was associated with a marked decrease in the risk of incident kidney stones (Taylor *et al.*, 2009). Dr Neil Barnard, president of the PCRM, states that animal protein is the worst kind of enemy of people with a tendency towards kidney stones or any kidney disease (Barnard, 1998). The animal protein in red meat, poultry, fish, eggs and milk tend to overwork the kidneys causing their filtering abilities to decline. This may make matters worse in a person who already has kidney disease. Additionally, animal protein causes calcium to be leached from the bones and excreted in the urine, adding further to the burden on the overworked kidney.

A report published in the Lancet in 1992 suggested that soya products may be beneficial in kidney disease. Kidney disease patients with protein in the urine and high cholesterol levels were placed on a cholesterol-free, low-protein, low-fat, high-fibre vegetarian (vegan) diet containing soya products. The amount of protein excreted in the urine dropped considerably as did their blood cholesterol levels (D'Amico *et al.*, 1992). It was uncertain whether these results reflected the reduction in dietary protein and fat or if the favourable results arose from a change in the nature of the food consumed. Either way, switching from a diet containing meat and dairy products to a plant-based diet containing less fat and protein and more fibre was beneficial to patients with kidney disease.

In addition to avoiding animal protein in the diet, increasing the potassium intake has been shown to yield benefits as potassium reduces calcium excretion, which can decrease the risk of stone formation. Additionally, the beneficial effect of increasing the fluid intake and the subsequent dilution of urine is well known (Curhan *et al.*, 1993).

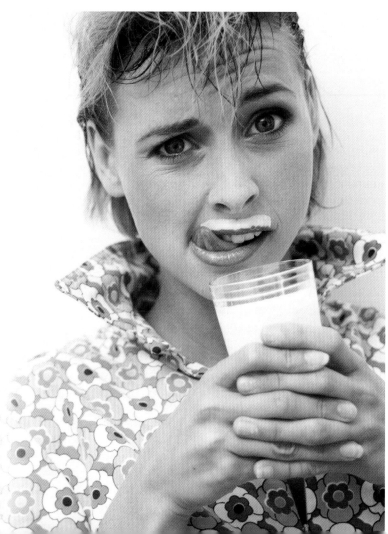

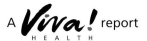

Lactose Intolerance

In 1836, after returning from the Beagle, Charles Darwin wrote "I have had a bad spell. Vomiting every day for eleven days, and some days after every meal." Darwin suffered for over 40 years from long bouts of vomiting, stomach cramps, headaches, severe tiredness, skin problems and depression. A number of researchers now suggest that he suffered from lactose intolerance (Campbell and Matthews, 2005). His case is a good example of how easily lactose intolerance can be missed.

Lactose is a disaccharide made up from glucose and galactose. It is the primary carbohydrate (sugar) found exclusively in mammalian milk (Heyman, 2006). To obtain energy from lactose, it must be broken down to glucose and galactose by the enzyme lactase. This enzyme is found in the small intestine on the tips of the villi. Glucose and galactose are then readily absorbed into the bloodstream to provide energy. Lactose intolerance occurs when the body produces little or no lactase, or when the lactase it produces doesn't work. In the absence of lactase, lactose is fermented by bacteria in the large intestine. These bacteria produce hydrogen and a wide range of potential toxins (Matthews *et al.*, 2005).

Lactose intolerance and cow's milk allergy are often mistakenly confused. Lactose intolerance is caused by a lack of lactase, cow's milk allergy is an adverse immune reaction to proteins found in milk.

Hippocrates first described lactose intolerance around 400 years BC but the clinical symptoms have become recognised only in the last 50 years (Lomer *et al.*, 2008). Symptoms include diarrhoea, bloated and painful stomach and on some occasions nausea and vomiting. Typically lactose intolerance causes diarrhoea via an osmotic mechanism. However, persistent lactose-induced diarrhoea that lasts long after the lactose has gone may be caused by a signalling mechanism analogous to cholera or enterotoxin (Matthews *et al.*, 2005).

Other symptoms may include muscle and joint pain, headaches, dizziness, lethargy, difficulty with short-term memory, mouth ulcers, allergies (eczema, rhinitis, sinusitis and asthma) cardiac arrhythmia, sore throat, increased frequency of urination, acne and depression (Lomer *et al.*, 2008). The severity of symptoms depends on the level of lactase produced; someone producing moderate levels may experience mild symptoms, whereas a person producing very little or no lactase will suffer more severe symptoms. Even more worrying is that bacterial toxins may play a key role in several other diseases, such as diabetes, rheumatoid arthritis, multiple sclerosis and some cancers (Campbell *et al.*, 2009).

There are three types of lactase deficiency:

- Primary lactase deficiency (adult-type hypolactasia) is the most common form. In most mammals, lactase activity naturally declines at variable rates following weaning until it reaches undetectable levels (Lomer, 2008). Generally the age of onset ranges from 1-20 years (Rasinperä *et al.*, 2004). However, it is not unknown for lactose intolerance to develop in people over 20 (Seppo *et al.*, 2008).
- Secondary (acquired) lactase deficiency is caused by illness, injury or medication. It can result from digestive diseases of the small intestine (such as ulcerative colitis and Crohn's disease), or intestinal damage caused by infections (such rotavirus and Giardia) (Matthews, 2005). Chemotherapy and long courses of antibiotics can cause lactose intolerance too. This may be temporary, but if caused by a long-term condition, could be permanent.
- Congenital lactase deficiency is an extremely rare disorder of new-borns associated with a complete absence of lactase. Affected infants present with intractable diarrhoea as soon as human milk or lactose-containing formula is introduced. Infants with this condition would not be expected to survive before the 20th century, as no suitable lactose-free formula was available (Heyman, 2006).

For some years, it was thought that lactase persistence in humans was the 'wild-type' pattern. It is now widely accepted that in adulthood, lactase deficiency is the normal state for most people (Lomer *et al.*, 2008). A staggering 4,000 million people cannot digest lactose properly (Campbell *et al.*, 2009). In fact, around 70 per cent of the world's population has primary lactase deficiency (Heyman, 2006; Lomer *et al.*, 2008). It is most prevalent in Asian and African countries with 80-100 per cent frequency. In Northern Europe, prevalence varies between one and 18 per cent (Rasinperä, 2004). The age of onset varies among different ethnic populations. Around 20 per cent of Hispanic, Asian and black children under five show some evidence of lactase deficiency (Heyman, 2006), while low lactase levels are rarely seen in white children under five (Rasinperä, 2004.

The widespread prevalence of lactose intolerance suggests that lactase deficiency is the normal or natural state and that the ability to continue to digest lactose after weaning originates from a genetic mutation that provided a selective advantage to populations using dairy products (Swagerty et al., 2002). This idea is supported by William Durham in his book Coevolution (Durham, 1991). Durham describes milk as baby food not 'intended' for adult consumption. He describes how the ability to digest lactose is the exception to the norm and can originally be traced back to a minority of pastoral tribes: the Tutsi and Hutu of Rwanda; the Fulani of West Africa; the Sindhi of North India; the Tuareg of West Africa and some European tribes. People who have retained the normal intolerance of lactose include: Chinese, Japanese, Inuit, native Americans, Australian Aborigines, Iranians, Lebanese and many African tribes including the Zulus, Xhosas and Swazis. These people, generally, do not have a history of pastoralism. As stated in Part One (The Origins of Dairy Farming) lactase persistence only developed around 8,000 years ago. In evolutionary terms, this is very recent history.

A range of tests can be used to diagnose lactose intolerance. The breath hydrogen test is currently considered to be the most cost-effective, non-invasive reliable test (Lomer et al., 2006). However, it involves drinking a lactose solution and can cause severe symptoms, sometimes lasting for days (Matthews, 2005). In rare cases a small bowel biopsy may be used to measure lactase levels. However, this invasive technique is usually used to determine whether the symptoms are caused by another condition, such as coeliac disease. A stool acidity test may be used to check infants for lactose intolerance. This is because large doses of lactose, such as those given in the breath hydrogen test, are dangerous for young children. Also, infants are more likely to develop dehydration caused by diarrhoea. DNA analysis of blood samples could offer a quick and easy to way to diagnose lactose intolerance and may help to differentiate patients with primary and secondary lactase deficiency (Lomer et al., 2008). However, this test is not yet routinely available.

When a dairy exclusion diet appears to fail, lactose intolerance is often mistakenly ruled out (Matthews et al., 2005). This is because lactose is added to many unexpected (non-dairy) foods and may continue producing symptoms in a patient convinced they are on a lactose-free diet. Lactose is used as a browning agent in bread and cakes, it is added to

processed meats (sausages and burgers) and even injected into some chicken meat. It is also added to some soft drinks and lagers. Breakfast drinks, powders and slimming products can contain as much lactose as cow's milk and it is often used in sauces supplied to butchers and restaurants (Matthews et al., 2005). Since 25 November 2005, all pre-packed foods sold in the UK have to show clearly on the label if they contain milk or any of the ingredients of milk.

Treatment depends on how sensitive the patient is to lactose. If they are mildly intolerant, they may be able to tolerate small amounts of some dairy foods. Fermented dairy foods (such as probiotic yoghurt and milk, sour cream, cottage cheese and hard cheeses, such as Edam and Cheddar) contain less lactose than fresh dairy products. Alternatively lactase may be taken in liquid form or capsules before a meal or added to cow's milk. Low lactose milk is also available in supermarkets but is quite sweet as it contains galactose and glucose from degraded lactose. Other animal milks (such as goat's milk), are not lactose-free. In fact, the lactose content of goat's and cow's milk are very similar; goat's milk contains 4.4g of lactose per 100g and whole milk contains 4.5g per 100g and semi-skimmed contains 4.7g per 100g (FSA, 2002). Of course, non-dairy products (such as soya, rice and oat milk) are excellent alternatives that do not require any monitoring at all.

Avoiding all lactose means cutting out all dairy foods and checking labels for lactose in bread, chocolate and other processed foods including meats. In addition, lactose is used in some types of medication so the patient should check with their GP or pharmacist (although symptoms of lactose intolerance rarely occur as a result of taking medication containing it).

Although there is no evidence of calcium deficiency in people eating a Chinese or Japanese diet with no lactose (Matthews, 2005), patients cutting out dairy foods may need some help and advice on how to ensure they still get plenty of calcium. This may be important for young children who need calcium for healthy growth and development. There are many excellent non-dairy sources of calcium including non-oxalate dark green leafy vegetables (broccoli, kale, spring greens, cabbage, bok choy and watercress), dried fruits (figs and dates), nuts (almonds and Brazil nuts) and seeds (sesame seeds and tahini, which contains a massive 680 milligrams

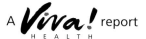

of calcium per 100 grams) (FSA, 2002). The dairy industry frequently cites the poor absorption of calcium from spinach as an example of how 'superior' cow's milk is as a source of calcium. However, spinach is an unusually poor source of calcium compared to other plant foods as it contains higher levels of oxalate which binds calcium and lowers its availability. Pulses (soya beans, kidney beans, chick peas, baked beans, broad beans, lentils, peas and calcium-set tofu) also provide a good source, as does calcium-fortified soya milk.

Although rarely life-threatening, the symptoms of lactose intolerance can lead to significant discomfort, disrupted quality of life, loss of school attendance and leisure and sports activities and work time, all at a cost to individuals, families and society (Heyman, 2006). The terminology relating to lactose intolerance (as opposed to milk protein allergy) can be confusing. It is therefore crucial to ensure that these problematic terms do not cause diagnostic mistakes and inappropriate treatment (Harrington and Mayberry, 2008).

In conclusion, drinking cow's milk is neither normal nor natural. The health implications of being the only mammal to consume milk as adults (and not just that, milk from another species too) are becoming clearer in the scientific literature as levels of the so-called diseases of affluence soar. The treatment for lactose intolerance is straightforward: avoid lactose. This means cutting out all dairy foods and checking labels for lactose in bread, chocolate and other processed foods.

Migraine

A migraine is much more than a bad headache; unless you suffer from them it is difficult to appreciate just how debilitating a migraine can be. Often people with a migraine can do nothing but lie quietly in a darkened room waiting for the pain to pass. The pain is excruciating, often accompanied by nausea, vomiting and an increased sensitivity to light and sound. A migraine can last for a few hours or a few days. Migraines occur more commonly in women than men (one in four women and one in 12 men) in the UK. and usually affect people in their teenage years up to around 40 years of age, although they do sometimes occur in children. Migraine affects about 15 per cent of adults in the UK (NHS Choices, 2012q).

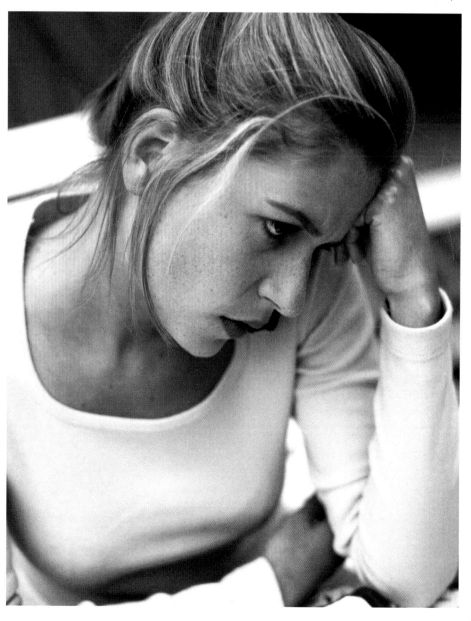

A range of common factors that can cause migraines in some people have been identified. Some scientists suggest that fluctuating levels of hormones may be linked to the causes of migraines (hence the higher number of women affected). Other factors include: emotional, physical, environmental, medicinal and dietary factors. Foods are frequently identified as triggers and the most common culprits include dairy products (particularly cheese), chocolate, alcohol (particularly red wine), caffeine, citrus fruits, nuts, fried foods and foods containing monosodium glutamate (MSG) such as some Chinese food, processed meats and frozen pizzas. Other triggers include cigarette smoke, bright lights, hunger, certain drugs (such as sleeping tablets, HRT and the combined oral contraceptive pill), loud noises, strong smells, neck and back pain, stress and tiredness. All these factors and others can lead to a migraine, and some people may experience a migraine following any one or a combination of these factors.

One study looked at a range of 36 possible (hormonal, environmental and dietary) triggering factors that may precipitate a migraine in a group of 123 migraine sufferers. The dietary factors included: chocolate, cheese, citrus fruits, alcohol, aspartame, MSG, a fat-rich diet, dairy products and caffeine as well as skipped meals or fasting and deprivation or insufficient intake of water. Out of all the patients tested, only 2.4 per cent did not complain about any dietary factor (Camboim Rockett *et al.*, 2012). The national medical charity Allergy UK lists cheese (particularly Stilton, Brie, Camembert and Emmenthal) as the third commonest cause of food-induced migraine after alcohol and chocolate. They suggest that 29 per cent of food-induced migraines are caused by alcohol, 19 per cent by chocolate, 18 per cent by cheese and 11 per cent by citrus foods. Other foods thought to trigger migraine include fried and fatty foods, onions, pork, pickled herring and yeast extract (Allergy UK, 2005).

In a study at Great Ormond Street Children's Hospital in London, 88 children with severe and frequent migraines were treated with a diet that eliminated many foods linked to migraine, 93 per cent of the children responded well to the diet and were free of headaches (Egger *et al.*, 1983). Foods were gradually reintroduced to identify those most likely to provoke a migraine. Top of the list was cow's milk, followed by chocolate (containing cow's milk), the food preservative benzoic acid, eggs, the synthetic yellow food colouring agent tartrazine, wheat, cheese, citrus, coffee and fish. Interestingly, children who

had initially developed a migraine in response to factors other than food (for example flashing lights or exercise) no longer responded to these triggers while on the special elimination diet.

The relationship between food allergy or intolerance and migraine is difficult to prove and, despite the evidence, remains a controversial subject. However, the possibility of cow's milk allergy or intolerance should be considered in all cases of migraine.

Multiple sclerosis and autoimmunity

Multiple sclerosis (MS) is the most common disease of the central nervous system (the brain and spinal cord) affecting young adults in the UK. It is estimated that there are currently around 100,000 people with MS in the UK. Symptoms usually first develop between the ages of 15 and 45, with the average age of diagnosis being about 30. For reasons that are unclear, MS is twice as common in women than men and more common in white people than black and Asian people (NHS Choices, 2012r).

Sclerosis means scarring and multiple refers to the different sites at which the scarring can occur throughout the brain and spinal cord. In MS the protective sheath (myelin) that surrounds the nerve fibres of the central nervous system becomes damaged. When myelin is damaged (demyelination) the messages between the brain and other parts of the body become disrupted. Myelin protects the nerve fibres in much the same way that household electrical wires are protected by an insulating cover. If this cover becomes damaged the normal signalling route becomes disrupted and may result in a short-circuit. The severity of the symptoms depends on how much damage has occurred to the central nervous system. More severe symptoms include blurred vision, paralysis, slurred speech, lack of coordination and incontinence.

Around eight out of 10 people with MS will have a type of MS called 'relapsing-remitting'. This means they will have periods of remission (that can last for days, weeks or even months) where symptoms are mild or disappear altogether. Remission is followed by a flare-up of symptoms, known as a relapse, which can last from a few weeks to few months. Usually after around 10 years, around half of people with relapsing-remitting MS go on to develop

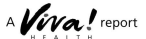

secondary progressive MS whereby symptoms gradually worsen and there are fewer or no periods of remission. The least common form of MS is primary progressive MS in which symptoms gradually get worse over time and there are no periods of remission (NHS Choices, 2012r). A subgroup of patients with relapsing-remitting MS exhibits a benign course with no disease progression and minimal disability decades after the first manifestations. Eventually, these patients may switch to a progressive state (Ramsaransing et al., 2009).

MS is an autoimmune disease whereby the body's immune system attacks its own tissues. As with other autoimmune diseases, it is thought that a combination of genetic factors and environmental triggers cause the disease. Recent research shows that an important environmental factor is diet (Ramsaransing et al., 2009). Other environmental triggers may include viruses or emotional factors such as stress. Interestingly, the incidence of MS increases the further you get from the equator, whether going north or south. For example, MS is relatively common in the UK, North America and Scandinavia, but rare in Malaysia or Ecuador. Campbell suggests that MS is over 100 times more prevalent in the far north than at the equator (Campbell and Campbell, 2005). In Australia the incidence of MS decreases seven-fold as you move towards the equator from the south to the north (Campbell and Campbell, 2005). This geographical distribution pattern applies to other autoimmune diseases including type 1 diabetes and rheumatoid arthritis (Campbell and Campbell, 2005). Indeed, this phenomenon has been noted since 1922 (Davenport, 1922). Campbell suggests in his book The China Study that autoimmune diseases should be considered as a group rather than as individual diseases as they share similar clinical backgrounds and sometimes occur in the same person or among the same populations (Campbell and Campbell,

2005). Interestingly, in the 1970s a correlation between the world distribution of dairy production and consumption and the incidence of multiple sclerosis was noted (Butcher, 1976). It was suggested then that dairy may be a contributing factor.

The research investigating the links between diet and MS dates back over 50 years to Dr Roy Swank's work first at the Montreal Neurological Institute in Norway, then at the Division of Neurology at the University of Oregon Medical School in the US. Swank was intrigued by the geographical distribution of MS and thought it may be due to dietary practices. Swank suspected animal foods high in saturated fats may be responsible as MS seemed to occur most among inland dairy-consuming populations and less among coastal fish-eating populations. Perhaps his best known trial was that published in the Lancet in 1990. In this study Swank followed 144 MS patients for a total of 34 years. Swank prescribed a low-saturated fat diet to all the participants but the degree of adherence to the diet varied widely. He observed how their conditions progressed. Results showed that for the group of patients who began the low-saturated fat diet (less than 20g per day saturated fat) during the earlier stages of MS, 95 per cent survived and remained physically active for approximately 30 years. Even those with significant disability were shown to markedly slow the progression of the disease if they could stick to the low-saturated fat diet. In contrast, 80 per cent of the patients with early-stage MS who did not adhere to the diet died of MS (Swank and Dugan, 1990). It was concluded that saturated animal fats increase the risk of MS.

Other studies have extended Swank's findings and revealed a positive correlation between the consumption of cow's milk and the incidence of MS. This later research suggests that there could be a combination of predisposing or precipitating factors involved in the aetiology of MS, and that environmental factors, such as the consumption of cow's milk, play a part (Agranoff *et al.*, 1974; Butcher, 1976). These and other studies suggest that cow's milk may contain some component other than saturated fat that influences the incidence of MS. For example, it has been suggested that this factor or environmental trigger may be a virus (Malosse *et al.*, 1992).

You are more likely to get MS if other people in your family have it (especially a brother or sister). This shows that there is an element of genetic predisposition in this disease. However, twin studies have shown that only about a quarter of identical twins with MS have a twin with the disease (Willer *et al.*, 2003). In other words for every four genetically identical sets of twins (one of whom has MS) one other twin will have the disease and three will not. If genes were solely responsible for MS, the genes that cause MS in one twin would also cause it in the other. When considering the role of genetics in a disease, it is also useful to look at what happens to the risk of that disease in migrating populations. As for cancer, heart disease and type 2 diabetes, people tend to acquire the MS risk of the population to which they move, especially if they move early in life. This shows that MS is more strongly related to environmental factors and diet than genes.

While the benefits of excluding milk from the diet may not have been directly proven for MS sufferers, there is evidence that a high intake of saturated fat increases the incidence and severity of this disease. Others studies suggest that increasing the intake of unsaturated fatty acids (such as linoleic acid), vitamin D and antioxidants may be helpful (Schwartz *et al.*, 2005). Recent studies concur that limiting the consumption of saturated fatty acid intake and supplementing with unsaturated fatty acids in combination with more vegetables can favour prognosis in relapsing-remitting MS (Ramsaransing *et al.*, 2009). This may be related to the anti-inflammatory properties of omega-3-fatty acids. This study also found that, compared to the daily recommended allowance, the MS patients studied had a lower than recommended intake of folic acid, magnesium, zinc and selenium. The overall message is clear: a plant-based diet low in fat, salt and sugar (and processed foods) and high in fresh fruits, vegetables, whole grains, pulses, nuts and seeds can provide all the vitamins, minerals and other nutrients required for good health and reduce some of the risk factors for MS or prevent making an already existing condition worse.

As the incidence of most autoimmune diseases correlates directly to the consumption of animal foods, this approach could help prevent other autoimmune conditions that occur increasingly among populations that consume high levels of dairy and meat products.

Overweight and obesity

Most people know what the term obesity means: an increased body weight caused by the excessive accumulation of fat. Overweight and obesity occur when more calories are taken into the body than are burnt up over time. In other words, if you don't burn up the energy you consume it will be stored as fat, and over time this may lead to excessive weight gain and obesity. So someone who works in a very physically demanding job, such as a building-site labourer, may need between 4,000 and 5,000 calories per day to maintain their normal weight. Whereas an office worker, who drives to work and does not take any exercise, may only need 1,500 calories per day.

Another way of defining obesity is to measure your body mass index (BMI). This is your weight in kilograms divided by the square of your height in metres. There are many websites that can do conversions and calculations for you (see Appendix II). In England, people with a body mass index between 25 and 29 are categorised as overweight, and those with an index of 30 or above are categorised as obese. If your BMI is over 40, you would be described as morbidly obese (NHS Choices, 2012s). The UK government describes 18.5 to 25 as healthy and suggests that a BMI of less than 18.5 is underweight. Alternatively, another useful method is to measure around your waist. People with very fat waists (94cm or more in men and 80cm or more in women) are more likely to develop obesity-related health problems (NHS Choices, 2012s).

Abdominal fat (also known as internal or visceral fat) is of particular concern because it's a key player in a variety of health problems including high blood pressure and cholesterol (which can lead to heart disease), diabetes and some cancers. You don't have to be overweight or obese to have high levels of this type of fat. Some slim people, who do little or no exercise, can have elevated levels of visceral fat. Unlike subcutaneous fat (the kind you can grasp with your hand), visceral fat lies deep within the abdominal region, hidden in the white fat that surrounds the vital

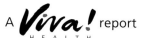

organs, streaked through underused muscles and wrapped around the heart. An MRI scan will reveal how much visceral fat a person has but from the outside it is impossible to tell. Hence the term 'tofi' – thin on the outside, fat on the inside. Such people are less likely to think they need to change their lifestyle and could unwittingly be at risk of serious health consequences. Research suggests that diet and exercise can be very effective in helping reduce visceral fat. Complex carbohydrates (fruits, vegetables and whole grains) and limiting the intake of simple carbohydrates such as white bread, white pasta and sugary drinks can help. Replacing saturated fats with polyunsaturated fats can also help.

In 2008, over a third (35 per cent) of all adults in the world were overweight, and more than one in ten (11 per cent) was obese. From 1980-2008, the worldwide prevalence of obesity nearly doubled with an estimated half a billion adults worldwide being described as obese. The highest levels of overweight and obesity occur in Canada, North and South America with 62 per cent overweight and 26 per cent obese. The lowest figures are seen in South East Asia (14 per cent overweight three per cent obese). In Europe, the Eastern Mediterranean and the Americas, over 50 per cent of women are overweight. For all three of these regions, roughly half of overweight women are obese (WHO, 2013d).

The main causes of obesity include an excessive intake of food coupled to a lack of exercise and a sedentary lifestyle. Other much less frequent causes include a genetic predisposition or an underlying illness (such as hypothyroidism). The British Medical Association (BMA) warns that childhood obesity levels have soared in the UK over recent years. They say that just over a quarter of adults in England are obese and three out of 10 children aged 2-15 in England are overweight or obese. **They warn that by 2050, it is estimated that half of the population in England will be obese** (BMA, 2013).

The BMA attribute this rise to the fact that children are eating too much for the

amount of physical activity they undertake. This is very worrying as early childhood obesity tends to indicate adult obesity which can lead to serious health risks later in life. Obesity is a known risk factor for many illnesses including type 2 diabetes, heart disease, high blood pressure, stroke, gall bladder disease and certain forms of cancer especially the hormonally related and large-bowel cancers. Childhood obesity is associated with a higher chance of obesity, premature death and disability in adulthood. But in addition to increased future risks, obese children experience breathing difficulties, increased risk of fractures, high blood pressure, early markers of CVD, insulin resistance and psychological effects (WHO, 2013e).

As populations become more urban and incomes rise, diets high in sugar, fat and animal products replace more traditional diets that were high in complex carbohydrates and fibre. Ethnic cuisine and unique traditional food habits are being replaced by westernised fast foods, soft drinks and increased meat consumption. Homogenisation and westernisation of the global diet has increased the energy density and this is particularly a problem for the poor in all countries who are at risk of both obesity and micronutrient deficiencies (Swinburn et al., 2004). This combined with a shift towards less physically demanding work, an increasing use of automated transport, technology in the home and more passive leisure pursuits means that people are less active than their parents and grandparents.

The WHO suggests several ways to lose weight including eating more fruit, vegetables, nuts and whole grains; engaging in daily moderate physical activity (60 minutes a day for children and 150 minutes per week for adults); cutting the amount of fatty, sugary foods in the diet and moving from saturated animal-based fats to unsaturated vegetable-oil based fats. Whole milk, cheese, cream, butter, ice-cream and most other dairy products, apart from skimmed and non-fat products, contain significant amounts of saturated fat and cholesterol. While we do need a certain amount of fat in the diet there is no nutritional requirement for saturated fat. Cow's milk is high in the unhealthy saturated fats and low in the healthy polyunsaturated essential fatty acids, which are required in the diet for good health. Most people eat much more fat than they need, and making minor changes to the diet (cutting down on fat) can make a big difference over time.

The Department of Health recommends that saturated fat should contribute no more than 11 per cent of the total energy that we get from food (Department of Health, 1991). Most people consume more than that. The 2012 National Diet and Nutrition Survey found that on average, saturated fat made up 12.8-13.6 per cent of food energy in all groups aged between four and 64 (Pot *et al.*, 2012). Compared with previous surveys, saturated fat intakes were somewhat lower in this study but, for adults, no statistically significant changes were observed. In general, the differences in absolute

intake of saturated fat were relatively small (1-3g per day). Clearly we are failing to heed the advice to reduce our intake of saturated fat.

Milk and dairy foods make a significant impact on saturated fat in the diet. Most saturated fat in the average UK diet comes from: milk, cheese, ice-cream, butter, margarine and fat-based spreads along with meat, pastry products (pies, tarts etc), bakery products (buns, biscuits, cakes), chocolate and chocolate confectionery and snacks. Approximately 65 per cent of the fat in milk is saturated and about three per cent of food energy is from dairy products making this a major target (Talbot, 2006).

A number of small-scale studies (of less than 35 obese adults) have suggested that the consumption of dairy products may actually help people lose weight (Zemel *et al.*, 2004; Zemel *et al.*, 2005). In these studies Professor Zemel, who has received a considerable amount of funding from the National Dairy Council, suggested that diets containing calcium from dairy foods might affect fat cell metabolism in such a way that greater weight loss can occur despite an identical calorie intake with a control group not consuming so much dairy.

The US National Dairy Council (who funded Zemel's research) is overseen by Dairy Management Incorporated, a non-profit corporation that defines its mission as increasing sales and demand for dairy products. Not dissimilar to the UK's dairy industry-funded DairyCo, Dairy Management Incorporated is funded by America's dairy farmers via a government-

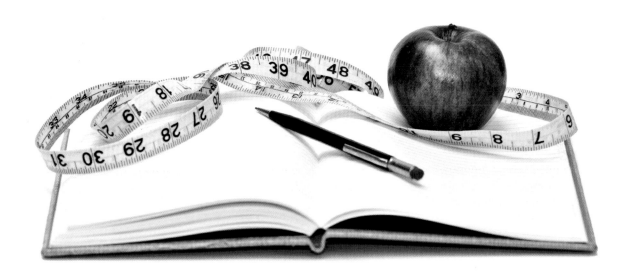

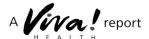

mandated fee. In 2009 they also received $5.3 million from the Agriculture Department to promote dairy sales overseas. In 2010, Dairy Management's annual budget approached a staggering $140 million. By comparison, the Center for Nutrition Policy and Promotion, which promotes healthy diets, had a total budget of just $6.5 million.

Dairy Management Incorporated has relentlessly marketed cheese despite the fact that Agriculture Department data show that cheese is a major reason the average US diet contains too much saturated fat. They employed a whole new marketing strategy with a weight-loss campaign based on Zemel's research. However, a subsequent study (by a research group including Zemel but not as the first named author) found no evidence that a diet high in dairy products enhances weight loss (Thompson *et al*., 2005). Furthermore, research that they also hoped would support Zemel's work found no evidence of dairy-related weight loss (Harvey-Berino *et al*., 2005). Dairy Management Incorporated pressed on with its advertising campaign regardless.

Dr Amy Lanou, the nutrition director of the PCRM, warned that care should be taken when interpreting the findings from Zemel's trials. Furthermore, Lanou suggested that the US National Dairy Council's claims promoting dairy consumption for weight loss went well beyond Zemel's findings. Lanou suggests that it was likely that calorie restriction, not dairy consumption, caused the weight loss reported in these studies (Lanou, 2005).

In June 2005 the PCRM decided enough was enough and filed two separate lawsuits to stop the multimillion-dollar advertising campaign claiming that milk facilitates weight loss. They filed one lawsuit to the US Food and Drugs Administration and the other to the US Federal Trade Commission. In the lawsuit the PCRM charged the National Dairy Council, the International Dairy Foods Association, Dairy Management Incorporated, Dannon Company, Kraft Foods and other dairy manufacturers with purposefully misleading customers (PCRM, 2005). Astonishingly, government lawyers defended the campaign, saying that the Agriculture Department reviewed, approved and continually oversaw the effort. Dr Walter C. Willett, chairman of the nutrition department at the Harvard School of Public Health and a former member of the federal government's nutrition advisory committee, said: "The USDA should not be involved in these programs that are promoting foods that we are consuming too much

of already. A small amount of good-flavoured cheese can be compatible with a healthy diet, but consumption in the U.S. is enormous and way beyond what is optimally healthy".

The dairy industry's national advertising campaign promoting the notion that people could lose weight by consuming more dairy products went on for a total of four years finally ending in 2007 when the Federal Trade Commission acted on the two-year-old petition by the PCRM. The Agriculture Department and dairy officials agreed to halt the campaign pending further research. Dairy Management Incorporated moved on to promoting milk and dairy foods in other areas such as promoting chocolate milk in schools and encouraging companies like Domino's pizza to use even more cheese in its pizzas (Domino's Wisconsin pizza now has six cheeses on top and two more in the crust). In an article in the *New York Times*, Dr Neal D. Barnard, president of the PCRM said: "If you want to look at why people are fat today, it's pretty hard to identify a contributor more significant than this meteoric rise in cheese consumption" (Moss, 2010). This may seem little to do with overweight and obesity problems in the UK, but these issues are mirrored here and trends show that we are not that far behind the extreme levels of obesity seen in the US.

Despite the dairy industry's claims outlined above, scientific studies show that adding dairy products to the diet does not help control weight; in fact the research confirms that in many cases the reverse is true, consuming milk and dairy foods can lead to weight gain. Some studies designed to test the effects of dairy consumption on weight found no difference in weight between groups consuming relatively large amounts of dairy foods compared to groups consuming little (Lappe *et al*., 2004; Gunther *et al*., 2005). Another study, this time of the effects of just calcium supplementation on weight loss in women who had recently given birth, found no relationship between calcium supplementation and weight loss (Wosje, 2004). Researchers at the University of British Columbia in Vancouver, Canada, who reviewed the scientific literature on the effects of dairy products or calcium supplements on body weight found that out of nine studies on dairy products, seven showed no significant difference while two studies linked weight gain to dairy consumption (Barr *et al*., 2003). Furthermore, out of 17 studies on calcium supplementation, just one reported weight loss. The authors state that interpreting such findings is limited by the inability to accurately determine the extent of compensation for the energy intake from the added dairy products. In other words, people who increased their dairy intake may have maintained the same energy intake (and so not gained weight) by reducing other foods. For example, the authors of one of the studies reviewed noted that the dairy product group in their study may have reduced their consumption of baked goods to compensate for the additional intake of dairy foods. Furthermore serious questions have arisen regarding the ability of diet records to reflect actual energy intake.

Another large scale study that followed over 12,000 children for three years concluded that the children who drank the most milk gained the most weight (Berkey et al., 2005). The analyses showed that out of milk, calcium, dairy fat and total energy intake, it was energy intake that was the most important predictor of weight gain. The authors attribute this weight to... you've guessed it, the added calories!

On the other hand, numerous studies show that a low-fat plant-based diet can be very effective in helping lose and maintain a healthy weight (Turner-McGrievy et al, 2007; Barnard et al., 2009). A recent study looked at the effects of eating a low-fat plant-based diet for 18 weeks on body weight and CVD risk in people with a BMI of 25 or higher and/or a previous diagnosis of type 2 diabetes. Results showed the average weight loss was 2.9 kg (compared to 0.06 kg in the control group). Total and LDL ('bad') cholesterol also fell in the test group. It was concluded that dietary intervention using a low-fat plant-based diet improves body weight, plasma lipids and in individuals with diabetes, it can also help control blood sugar levels (Mishra et al., 2013).

To most people it is just common sense, a calorie is a calorie and weight gain or weight loss is a case of mathematics. If you take in more energy (calories) than you use, you will gain weight. If you use up more energy than you consume, you will lose weight. There is no magic bullet, and if there were it seems very unlikely that it would be cow's milk, butter or cheese.

Osteoporosis

Osteoporosis (meaning porous bones) is a condition that affects the bones, causing them to become weak and more likely to fracture. Although the whole skeleton is usually affected, fractures most commonly occur in the spine, wrist and hips (NHS Choices, 2012t). Osteoporosis is sometimes called the silent disease as there are often no symptoms until a fracture occurs.

Bones consist of a thick outer shell and a strong inner mesh filled with a protein called collagen, calcium salts and other minerals. Osteoporosis occurs when calcium is lost from the bones and they become more fragile and prone to fracture. This debilitating condition tends to occur mostly in postmenopausal women between 51 and 75 due to a lack of the hormone oestrogen, which helps to regulate the incorporation of calcium into the bones. It can occur earlier or later and not all women are at equal risk of developing osteoporosis. Around three million people in the UK are thought to have osteoporosis and there are over 250,000 fractures every year as a result. Although commonly associated with post-menopausal women, osteoporosis can also affect men, younger women and children (NHS Choices, 2012t). In the UK, one in two women and one in five men over the age of 50 will break a bone mainly because of poor bone health (National Osteoporosis Society, 2013).

Osteoporosis has been called the silent epidemic as the first sign some people experience is a fracture. In 2006, the dairy industry responded to this health scare by promoting milk, cheese and yogurt directly to teenage girls in an advertising campaign called Naturally Beautiful, run by the Milk Development Council with the support from the European Commission (MDC, 2005a). Since then, the promoting of cow's milk and cheese to teenage girls for bone health has decreased. DairyCo now tends to focus more on promoting milk in schools by providing 'educational resources' and website material for schools as well as promoting dairy farming actively to the public through their consumer facing website as well as talking to the media (Dairy Co, 2013d). Most people know about osteoporosis and it is commonly assumed that dairy products can help protect against it. Indeed it is deeply entrenched in the British psyche that calcium from dairy sources is essential for good bone health. However, this association is more to do with successful marketing than scientific evidence.

In 2012, researchers from The WHO Collaborating Centre for Metabolic Bone Diseases, at the University of Sheffield Medical School in the UK published a review of hip fracture incidence and probability of fracture worldwide. Figure 9.0 shows the hip fracture

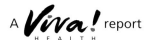

Figure 9.0 World age-standardised hip fracture rates for women per 100,000 in selected countries.

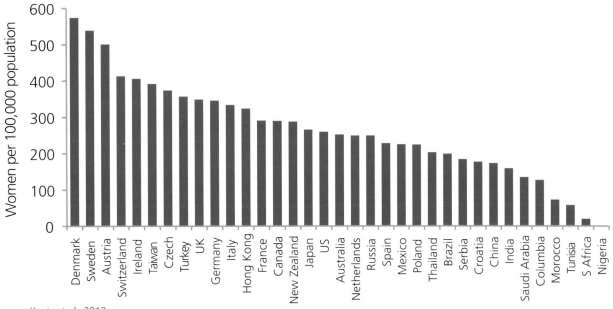

Source: Kanis *et al*., 2012.

rates for women per 100,000 from a range of countries. The pattern for men was broadly similar to that for women. The authors of this review observed a greater than 10-fold variation in hip fracture risk between countries (Kanis *et al*., 2012). The high-risk countries extended from North Western Europe (Iceland, UK, Ireland, Denmark, Sweden and Norway) through central Europe (Belgium, Germany, Austria, Czech Republic, Slovakia, Hungary, Switzerland and Italy) to the south east (Greece, Slovenia) and onwards (to the Lebanon, Oman and Iran). Other high-risk countries for women were Hong Kong, Singapore, Malta and Taiwan. Notably, if ethnic-specific rates were considered in the US, then Hispanic, Asian and Black populations (often lactose intolerant and so non-milk consumers) would be described as low risk but Caucasian women were deemed to be at a high risk (this is why the US appears in the middle of the graph). Regions of moderate risk included Oceania (a region centred on the islands of the tropical Pacific Ocean), the Russian Federation, the southern countries of Latin America and the countries of North America. Low-risk regions included the northern regions of Latin America, Africa, Jordan and Saudi Arabia, India, China, Indonesia and the Philippines. In Europe, the majority of countries were categorised at high or moderate risk with the exceptions of Croatia and Romania (Kanis *et al*., 2012).

In summary, fracture rates are highest in Caucasian women living in temperate climates and are somewhat lower in women from Mediterranean and Asian countries and are lowest among women in Africa. Countries in economic transition, such as Hong Kong, have seen significant increases in fracture rates in recent decades (WHO, 2003a). This indicates that environmental factors, such as diet, may be responsible. This view is supported by

changes in risk in immigrant populations. For example, black Americans have a lower fracture risk than Caucasians in the US, but a much higher risk than black Africans. A similar scenario is seen among the Japanese population of Hawaii compared to those in Japan and Chinese people living in Singapore compared with mainland China (Kanis *et al*., 2012).

Many risk factors for osteoporosis have been identified including a low body mass index (BMI), low bone mineral density, reduced sunlight exposure (crucial for vitamin D production in the skin), early menopause, smoking, alcohol consumption and low physical activity levels. In addition, somewhat unexpectedly, obesity has been identified as a risk factor; so being underweight or overweight can increase the risk. Migration status obesity (whereby obesity levels among migrants are significantly higher compared with the native population as a result of increased availability of poor quality food and/or increased exposure to aggressive marketing of fast food), is also a risk factor (Kanis *et al*., 2012). Numerous dietary factors are thought to influence bone health and fracture risk, including: calcium, vitamin D, protein (including the ratio of plant to animal protein), potassium, sodium and fruit and vegetables (Appleby *et al*., 2007). Assessing the relative contribution of each of these is difficult as nutrients are not consumed in isolation and may work together or be influenced by other factors. Furthermore the experimental data is somewhat inconsistent with conflicting findings.

Figure 9.0 supports earlier research that shows how Western style diets accompany hip fracture rates around the world. There are a number of theories as to why this could be. One of the most popular - and controversial - is the acid-alkaline hypothesis.

The acid-alkaline hypothesis

The hypothesis that a high animal protein diet could be a risk factor for osteoporosis dates back to research conducted more than 40 years ago (Barzel and Jowsey, 1969). The hypothesis proposes that as food is digested, acids are released into the blood, and the body attempts to neutralise the acid by drawing calcium from the bones. This calcium is then excreted in the urine (the calciuric response). Animal proteins, from cow's milk and dairy products, meat, fish and eggs, are said to have a particularly bad effect because of the greater amount of sulphur-containing amino acids they contain compared to most plant proteins. Sulphur-containing amino acids give rise to sulphuric acid when they are broken down in metabolism.

Modern diets in industrialised countries are considerably more acid-forming than the more alkalising foods that would have been consumed throughout the vast majority of human evolution. Just consider a beef-burger in a white bun with fries and a fizzy drink compared to nuts, seeds, fruit, leaves and water with the occasional piece of meat and/or fish… Consequently, it is suggested that humans may be poorly adapted to the contemporary acid-forming diets and that this may contribute to modern epidemics of chronic disease (Scialla and Anderson, 2013).

Until relatively recently, the acid-alkaline hypothesis has been widely accepted; in 2003, in their recommendations for preventing osteoporosis, the WHO stated that:

"With regard to calcium intakes to prevent osteoporosis, the Consultation referred to the recommendations of the Joint FAO/WHO Expert Consultation on Vitamin and Mineral Requirements in Human Nutrition which highlighted the calcium paradox. The paradox (that hip fracture rates are higher in developed countries where calcium intake is higher than in developing countries where calcium intake is lower) clearly calls for an explanation. To date, the accumulated data indicate that the adverse effect of protein, in particular animal (but not vegetable) protein, might outweigh the positive effect of calcium intake on calcium balance." WHO, 2003a.

A substantial body of evidence links animal protein to a decrease in bone mineral density. A study, looking at hip fracture incidence in 33 different countries in relation to consumption of plant and animal protein, found that the countries with the lowest fracture rates also had the lowest intakes of animal protein. Conversely, in 10 of the 11 countries with the highest fracture rates, animal protein intake exceeded plant protein intake. The authors said that hip fracture incidence is directly related to animal protein intake and suggested that bone integrity is compromised by acid that results from the metabolism of animal proteins. They suggested that the moderation of animal food intake, coupled to an increased ratio of vegetable to animal food consumption, may confer a protective effect (Frassetto et al., 2000). Another study of 1,035 elderly women found that women with a high ratio of animal to vegetable protein intake had a greater risk of hip fracture than those with a low ratio (Sellmeyer et al., 2001). A further study of 757 young girls in urban Beijing in China, compared the effects of protein intakes from animal and plant sources on bone mass accrual over five years. Results showed that protein from animal foods, particularly meat, had negative effects on bone mineral content. It was concluded that higher protein intake, especially from animal foods, has a significant negative effect on bone mass accrual in pre-pubertal girls (Zhang et al., 2010).

Another study compared the effects of animal and plant protein in the diets of overweight and obese post-menopausal women dieting. They found that the energy-restricted diet with protein from meat sources promoted bone loss compared with an energy-restricted diet without meat. They concluded that for post-menopausal women, choosing a diet containing meat may decrease

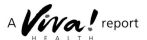

bone mineral density and increase the risk of osteoporosis (Campbell and Tang, 2010). This extends the findings of an earlier study which examined the levels of bone loss in 1,600 older women and found that vegetarians had lost only 18 per cent bone mineral compared to omnivores who had lost 35 per cent bone mineral by the age of 80 (Marsh *et al.*, 1988).

Cross-cultural studies summarising data on protein intake and fracture rates from 16 countries compared industrialised and non-industrialised lifestyles and revealed strong links between a high animal protein diet, bone degeneration and the occurrence of hip fractures (Abelow *et al.*, 1992). In the book The China Study, Campbell observed that in rural communities where animal protein made up just 10 per cent of the total protein intake (the other 90 per cent coming from plant-based sources) the bone fracture rate was one-fifth of that in the US where 50 per cent or more of total protein is made up of animal protein (Campbell and Campbell, 2005), again indicating a link between animal protein and bone degeneration. The traditional Inuit (or Eskimo) diet is made up almost entirely of animal protein. Inuits potentially have one of the highest calcium intakes in the world (up to 2,500 milligrams per day) depending on whether they eat whole fish, including the bones, or not. They also have a high rate of osteoporosis, even higher than white Americans (Mazess *et al.*, 1974; Mazess *et al.*, 1975; Pratt and Holloway, 2001).

A substantial body of evidence supports a positive link between fruit and vegetables and bone health. A review of the role of protein, calcium and bone health in women in the EPIC-Potsdam cohort in Germany found that vegetable protein played a positive role in maintaining good bone health (Weikhert *et al.*, 2005). Indeed, vegetable consumption was found to be an independent negative predictor for the worldwide incidence of hip fracture and high consumption of fruit and vegetables was positively associated with bone mineral density in both women and men (Weikhert *et al.*, 2005). The research showing that plant proteins confer a beneficial effect on bone health is consistent.

Other studies have investigated the effects of cow's milk and calcium in relation to bone health. The Harvard Nurses' Health study examined whether higher intakes of milk can reduce the risk of osteoporotic fractures. The study observed over 75,000 women for 12 years and concluded that

increasing milk consumption did not confer a protective effect against hip or forearm fracture. In fact the 1997 study found that an increased calcium intake from dairy foods was associated with a higher risk of fracture. They concluded that their results do not support the hypothesis that higher consumption of milk or other food sources of calcium by adult women protects against hip or forearm fractures (Feskanich *et al.*, 1997). In a 2003 follow-up of the Nurses' Health Study, the increased risk associated with dairy was not reported but they still found that higher daily intakes of cow's milk did not reduce the risk of hip fracture. In other words, there was still no evidence of a protective effect of dairy against fracture risk (Feskanich *et al.*, 2003). Interestingly, a lower risk of hip fracture was found among those with higher vitamin D intakes.

In a more recent extensive review of studies looking at total calcium intake and hip fracture risk, results showed that in prospective cohort studies, calcium intake was not significantly associated with hip fracture risk in women or men. The pooled results from randomised controlled trials not only found no reduction in hip fracture risk with calcium supplementation but suggested an increased risk with calcium supplementation among men and women (Bischoff-Ferrari *et al.*, 2007).

So, for children and adolescents, while an adequate intake of protein is necessary for good bone development and stability, some research suggests that large intakes of animal protein may counter this positive effect. In a study looking at long-term dietary protein intake, dietary acid load and bone status in children, it was concluded that the positive effect of protein could be negated, at least partly, by a high renal acid load. The authors say that their findings support the health benefit of a diet rich in alkali-yielding fruit and vegetables (which is in accordance with the 5-a-day campaign) and recommend an integrative approach saying that focusing on single nutrients is not sufficient (Alexy *et al.*, 2005). Such evidence, plus other studies showing that an animal protein-based diet (with the same total quantity of protein as a vegetarian diet) confers an increased risk for uric acid stones (Breslau *et al.*, 1988) have led some to suggest that the high calcium losses in the urine caused by animal protein may be a risk factor for the development of osteoporosis.

A number of studies, including observational epidemiology and some small clinical trials, have examined the role of the dietary acid load in people with chronic kidney disease. It has been suggested that the evidence largely supports the hypothesis of a direct relationship between a higher dietary acid load and chronic kidney disease progression, bone loss and sarcopenia (loss of skeletal muscle). However, due to a wide variety of techniques and terminology used to quantify the dietary acid load, this theory is not widely appreciated by nephrologists (Scialla and Anderson, 2013). A number of critical reviews of the acid-alkaline hypothesis have been published (Darling *et al*., 2009; Fenton *et al*., 2009; Fenton *et al*., 2011). These reviews argue that a causal association between dietary acid load and osteoporosis is not supported by the research and say that there is no evidence that an alkaline diet can protect bone health (Fenton *et al*., 2011).

One of the main criticisms is that if bone is the primary source of calcium from which diet-related acid is buffered, it is suggested that all the bone in the body would be dissolved in just a few years (Bonjour, 2005). It is also argued that homeostatic mechanisms (including renal acid excretion) would not permit a steady-state low-grade metabolic acidosis caused by a typical Western diet. In other words, the body has ways of redressing the balance when, for example, the diet increases the acid levels in the blood, and even small increases in acidity are countered by these mechanisms – that is the theory anyway. However, it has been demonstrated that a high dietary acid load, which lies within the ranges seen in a typical American or European diet, can increase the acidity of blood to detectable levels (Frassetto and Sebastian, 2013). So, on the one hand we are told that we can compensate for the acidifying effects of a high-protein diet, while on the other hand, the research shows that we may not be able to balance it out completely. It may be that the truth lies somewhere between these two apparently irreconcilable arguments.

Buffers are chemical substances that can minimise changes in a liquid when it becomes more acidic or alkaline. To maintain equilibrium whilst there is an increased amount of acid in the body, at least three compensatory physiological responses are activated: buffering from the bone (and so some degree skeletal muscle), increased ventilation to eliminate carbon dioxide, and in the kidney, bicarbonate is generated and reabsorbed into the blood while excess hydrogen ions are secreted into the urine. In healthy people, these buffering systems all have a tremendous capacity to maintain the blood pH (acid-alkali balance) within a very narrow margin (Kerstetter, 2009). However, the major reservoir of alkali (in the form of alkaline salts of calcium) is the

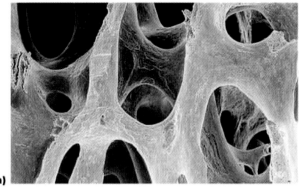

(a)
Normal bone

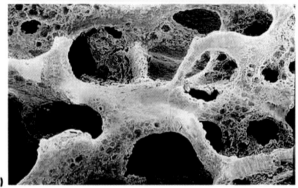

(b)
Osteoporotic bone

Image©2012 Midlands Technical College

skeleton, which provides the buffer needed to maintain blood pH and plasma bicarbonate concentrations (Pizzorno *et al*., 2010). While kidney metabolism represents a major mechanism by which metabolic acid loads are handled by the body, if the kidneys are overwhelmed or compromised (kidney function declines with age), calcium from the bones may be called on to compensate for the increasingly acidic environment and an alkalising diet could help redress the balance (Dargent-Molina *et al*., 2008; Frassetto and Sebastian, 2013). So, under certain conditions, the acid-alkaline hypothesis may provide a plausible mechanism in which a plant-based diet, rich in fruit and vegetables, could help promote and preserve bone health. This may go some way in explaining the apparently contradictory evidence concerning animal protein and bone health.

The acid-alkaline hypothesis has also been challenged on the basis of a series of short-term experimental studies that suggest that high-protein diets are not harmful to bone health and might actually be beneficial by improving calcium absorption (Kerstetter *et al*., 2003). However, while high-protein diets may increase calcium absorption, they also increase calcium excretion in the urine. Therefore, the positive effects of protein intake on bone health may only be beneficial under conditions of adequate calcium intake (Mangano *et al*., 2014). Indeed, growing evidence suggests that calcium and protein may interact in terms of bone health and that the potential harmful effect of a high-protein intake may be compensated for by an adequate calcium intake (Weikert *et al*., 2005). If there is insufficient calcium in the diet to counter the calciuric effect, calcium may be lost from the bone.

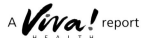

The generally accepted daily protein dietary allowance is 0.8g per kg of body weight. One study (of just 13 participants) compared a moderate animal protein intake to a high animal protein intake diet (1.0g per kg body weight compared to 2.1g per kg) and found with 800mg of calcium per day, all participants ended up in negative calcium balance (Kerstetter *et al.*, 2005). This was not anticipated and the authors suggested that the level of dietary calcium was not enough to maintain calcium balance. However, because the extra urinary calcium lost in the high-protein diet was found to come from the diet (as opposed to the bone), the authors concluded that, at least in the short term, high-protein diets are not detrimental to bone. While, the increased urinary calcium produced by the high protein diet may reflect enhanced calcium absorption and not bone resorption, under both the moderate and high protein diets tested, the vast majority (over 90 per cent) of the calcium found in the urine still came from the bones. Adult bones constantly undergo remodelling through bone resorption by osteoclasts and bone formation by osteoblasts. In adults, almost the entire human skeleton may be remodelled over a 10-year cycle. While this study suggests that higher protein intakes may not be harmful in the short term, it should be remembered that they can lead to kidney problems and increased levels of IGF-1 which are linked to certain cancers (see below). The long-term impact of high-protein diets on bone health is still unclear and the relative contribution of calcium from the bone and/or diet to protein-induced calciuria remains controversial (Heaney, 2002).

Other studies suggest that high-protein diets may increase calcium absorption and help preserve bone mass by stimulating IGF-1, a potent bone growth stimulator (Tang, 2014; Mangano *et al.*, 2014). However, as stated, increased IGF-1 levels are linked to an increased risk of certain cancers so high animal protein diets are therefore not desirable and should not be recommended (see IGF-1).

Results of observational epidemiological studies have not helped to clarify the nature of the effect of high-protein intakes on the skeleton (Dargent-Molina *et al.*, 2008). Some studies show a positive association with bone mass, some show no association and some show a negative association. Even fewer studies have investigated the effect of protein intake on fracture risk. These too have yielded mixed results including a decreased risk of fracture with higher protein intake, and increased risk of fracture with

Table 3.0 Potential acid as sulphate from sulphur-containing amino acids.

Food	mEq per g of protein
Oatmeal	0.82
Egg	0.80
Walnuts	0.74
Pork	0.73
Whole wheat	0.69
White rice	0.68
Barley	0.68
Tuna	0.65
Chicken	0.65
Corn	0.61
Beef	0.59
Cow's milk	0.55
Cheddar	0.46
Soya	0.40
Peanuts	0.40
Millet	0.31
Almonds	0.23
Potato	0.23

Source: Hoffman and Falvo, 2004.

higher protein and some studies identify proteins from animal sources as the key factor increasing fracture risk.

A further possible confounding factor is that it is commonly assumed that all animal proteins have a higher content of sulphur-containing amino acids than all plant proteins. However, this may not be entirely correct, some plant proteins (certain grains) may have a greater potential to produce more sulphuric acid than animal proteins (Massey, 2003). Medical professionals use milliequivalents (mEq) to measure electrolyte levels in body fluids. Table 3.0 shows the mEq of selected animal and plant foods and shows how some plant proteins may have a greater potential to produce more mEq of sulphuric acid per gram of protein than some animal proteins. For example, if protein comes from white rice it would have a mEq of 0.68 per gram of protein while protein from milk contains 0.55 mEq per gram of protein (Hoffman and Falvo, 2004).

As stated, this is a complex issue with a wide range of factors involved, not least the role of the kidney. It should be noted that people who consume a high-animal protein diet have an increased risk of kidney disease and continuing to consume high levels of meat, eggs and dairy foods may present a burden on an already overworked kidney (see Kidney Disease). It seems logical that the harder you make the kidneys work, the more likely they are to struggle to meet the challenge. There appears to be some consensus that in people with kidney disease or poor kidney function (resulting from aging), a high dietary acid load may result in acidosis which may then lead to bone and muscle loss. In a recent study looking at the effects of dietary acid load in chronic kidney disease it was concluded that in the setting of chronic kidney disease and aging, a higher dietary acid load (determined by the balance of acid-inducing foods such as meats, eggs, cheese and cereal grains against alkali-inducing foods such as fruits and vegetables) may result in low-grade, subclinical acidosis (Scialla and Anderson, 2013). The authors went on to say that in these circumstances, efforts to maintain stable blood pH and boost acid excretion from the kidney may lead to bone and muscle loss and further decline in kidney function, but that this may be mitigated by alkali. In summary, they say that studies with hard outcomes are needed to determine the degree of benefits of a foods-based approach to reducing the dietary acid load in patients with early to moderate chronic kidney disease.

The acid-alkaline hypothesis is a controversial area of research. Currently, data that support both the proponents and opponents of the acid-alkaline hypothesis exist (Frassetto and Sebastian, 2013). The pattern of incidence of osteoporosis around the world certainly suggests that some aspect of the typical Western lifestyle could be a significant contributing factor to bone loss. Furthermore, the evidence shows that animal protein can be harmful to bone health but clearly more research is required. In the meantime, it seems prudent to observe how the Western diet is accompanied by the so-called Western diseases including osteoporosis and limit, if not eliminate, all animal protein from the diet.

Calcium matters

If simply consuming sufficient levels of calcium was the answer to preventing bone loss, then Northwest European countries like Denmark, Sweden and the UK, and the US would have the lowest fracture rates in the world. This is simply not the case; in fact they have the highest rates, a fact that is often overlooked by health professionals. In the UK, the estimated average requirement (EAR) for calcium, whereby 50 per cent of the population's requirement is met, is set at 525mg per day. The recommended amount or reference nutrient intake (RNI), whereby 97.5 per cent of the population's requirement is met,

for calcium for adults is 700mg per day. The 2003 UK National Diet and Nutrition Survey found that the average calcium intake for men and women was 1,007mg and 777mg per day respectively (144 and 111 per cent of the RNI respectively). Younger adults tended to have lower intakes but these were still above the EAR of 525mg per day). Overall, men and women had significantly higher average daily intakes of calcium in the 2003 survey than in the 1986/87 Adults Survey (Henderson et al., 2003a). So while a relatively small number of people had intakes on the low side, generally, the level of calcium intake in the UK was good. If you are already getting enough calcium, just adding more isn't going to be helpful. It could be that getting sufficient calcium isn't the problem, but that holding on to it is. As stated, there are genetic and lifestyle factors that can cause calcium to be lost from the body.

It should be stated that very low calcium intakes have been linked to poor bone health. A large-scale EPIC-Oxford study found that women with a low calcium intake (less than 525mg per day) had an increased risk of bone fracture compared with women with a calcium intake of at least 1,200mg per day (Key et al., 2007). Another EPIC-Oxford study found that a higher fracture rate among vegans compared with meat-eaters was halved in magnitude by adjustment for energy and calcium intake and disappeared altogether when the analysis was restricted to subjects who consumed at least 525mg per day of calcium. In other words, there is no reason to believe that vegans who consume an adequate amount of calcium would have different bone fracture rates to vegetarians or meat-eaters. The authors concluded that an adequate calcium intake is essential for bone health, irrespective of dietary preferences (Appleby et al., 2007). In a more recent study, the average intake of calcium among a group of UK vegans was higher than in Appleby's 2007 study; 456 mg per day compared to 232 mg per day for men and 226 mg per day for women (Clarys et al., 2014). So, some people are not getting enough calcium in the diet and more care needs to be taken. This does not mean we should consume dairy products, far from it, the healthiest sources of calcium are plant-based foods that do not contain the harmful components found in cow's milk and dairy products. Furthermore, care should be taken not to consume too much calcium as high intakes may be linked to an increased risk of heart attack or stroke (Daly and Ebeling, 2010). The UK NHS suggests that taking 1,500mg or less a day is unlikely to cause any harm (NHS, 2012v).

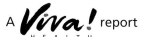

The role calcium plays in bone health is the hook the dairy industry uses to encourage parents to feed their children increasing amounts of dairy products. We have been repeatedly sold the line that cow's milk and dairy foods are the best source of calcium. However, while calcium remains important for bone health, it could be that focusing on achieving high levels of calcium (above recommended intakes) has little benefit and may even cause us to neglect other lifestyle factors that could offer greater benefits. A 2005 review on dairy products and bone health published in the official journal of the American Academy of Pediatrics concluded that there is very little evidence to support increasing the consumption of dairy products in children and young adults in order to promote bone health. This review examined the effects of dairy products and total dietary calcium on bone integrity in children and young adults and found that out of 37 studies, 27 showed no relationship between dairy or dietary calcium intake and measures of bone health. In the remaining studies the effects on bone health were either small or results were confounded by the fortification of milk with vitamin D (Lanou *et al.*, 2005). Another meta-analysis of 19 studies involving 2,859 children, published in the *British Medical Journal* found that calcium supplementation in children was unlikely to decrease the risk of fracture in childhood or in later life (Winzenberg *et al.*, 2006). In this analysis, there were few studies involving children with low intakes. It may be that, providing we get adequate calcium, supplementing the diet offers no benefit and may actually be detrimental.

This research strengthens previous evidence that extra calcium or and/or dairy products do not have a clinically relevant impact on bone health in youth. More recently, a prospective study involving 61,433 Swedish women followed over 19 years, investigated associations between the long-term dietary intake of calcium and risk of fracture and osteoporosis. The findings did show an association between very low dietary calcium intake and an increased risk of fractures but above the base level of 750mg, increased intakes of calcium were not associated with a reduction in risk of fracture or osteoporosis. In addition to that, the rate of hip fracture was actually increased in those with high dietary calcium intakes (Warensjö *et al.*, 2011).

Exercise

There are many factors linked to bone health that may be more important than calcium. For example, some studies show that exercise is the predominant lifestyle determinant of bone strength. When the bone density of 80 young women was monitored over a 10-year period, it showed that exercise was more important than calcium intake (Lloyd *et al.*, 2004). In a group of older people, a 15-year investigation into whether low calcium intake was a risk factor for hip fractures concluded that cutting back on dairy did not increase the risk and that physical activity provided better protection (Wickham *et al.*, 1989). The discovery of 18th-century human bones under a London church revealed that today's women lose far more calcium than our ancestors (Lees *et al.*, 1993). This may be attributed to the lower degree of physical activity undertaken today. This research supports an increasing amount of evidence that physical activity is a key factor in reducing osteoporosis risk.

Salt

Other studies suggest a detrimental effect of dietary salt (sodium chloride) on bone health. One study describes how a typical American diet contains amounts of sodium chloride far above evolutionary norms and potassium levels far below. This imbalance is thought to contribute to the acid producing effects of a typical Western diet. This may contribute to development of osteoporosis, kidney stones and other health problems. The authors point out how, after seven million years of hominid evolution, humans remain genetically adapted to the potassium-rich, sodium-chloride-poor, alkali-producing diet of our ancestral hunter-gatherers. In other words, our bodies are not well-suited to an acid-producing diet. The shift to the contemporary diet occurred too recently for evolutionary forces to have had the opportunity to make any changes in our metabolic machinery. However, they suggest that decreasing salt intake and increasing the intake of plant foods may not just help the aging skeleton but provide other potential health benefits as well (Frassetto *et al.*, 2008).

Vitamin K

Other studies suggest a positive role in bone health for vitamin K. A review of projects funded by the UK Food Standards Agency examined the potential benefits of fruit and vegetables, vitamin K, early-life nutrition and vitamin D on bone health. They reached two conclusions; firstly that a diet rich in fruit and vegetables might be beneficial to bone health and secondly that an increased consumption of vitamin K may also contribute to bone health. A major research gap they identified was the need to investigate vitamin D status in relation to bone health in different groups (Ashwell *et al.*, 2008). A higher calcium intake is still the primary recommendation for the prevention of osteoporosis, and vitamin D deficiency is often overlooked. In a study of US adults, a large proportion of younger and older adults were found to be below the desirable vitamin D threshold, whereas calcium intakes seemed to be adequate in the majority of individuals. The authors concluded that the correction of vitamin D status is more important than increasing dietary calcium intake (Bischoff-Ferrari *et al.*, 2009).

The idea that humans must suckle from cows for their entire lives in order to meet their calcium needs is clearly absurd. An increasing amount of evidence now shows that milk is not the best source of calcium at all and suggests that our bone health would benefit enormously if we switched to plant-based sources. Interestingly, the 2003 National Diet and Nutrition Survey showed that a large share of the calcium in our diets (over 50 per cent) comes from sources other than dairy foods (Henderson *et al.*, 2003a). This is not surprising as most people in the world (over 70 per cent) obtain their calcium from plant-based sources rather than dairy products. Good plant-based sources of calcium include non-oxalate dark green leafy vegetables such as broccoli, kale, spring greens, cabbage, bok choy and watercress. Also rich in calcium are dried fruits, such as figs and dates, nuts, particularly almonds and Brazil nuts, and seeds including sesame seeds and tahini (sesame seed paste) which contains a massive 680mg of calcium per 100g. Pulses including soya beans, kidney beans, chick peas, baked beans, broad beans, lentils, peas

and calcium-set tofu (soya bean curd) provide a good source of calcium. A good additional source is calcium-enriched soya milk. Interestingly, the calcium in dairy products is not as well absorbed as that in many dark green leafy vegetables, for example, in one study, calcium absorbability from kale was demonstrated to be considerably higher than that from cow's milk (Heaney and Weaver, 1990).

The interaction between calcium intake and physical activity, sun exposure/vitamin D, intake of vitamin K, sodium, protein and protective phytonutrients (soya compounds), needs to be considered before recommending increased calcium intake in countries with low fracture incidence (WHO, 2003a). In a paper in the British Medical Journal, Dr Amy Lanou suggests that it is time to revise our calcium recommendations for young people and change our assumptions about the role of calcium, milk and other dairy products in the bone health of children and adolescents. Lanou argues that while the policy experts work on revising recommendations, doctors and other health professionals should encourage children to spend time in active play or sports and to consume a nutritious diet built from whole foods from plant sources to achieve and maintain a healthy weight and provide an environment conducive to building strong bones (Lanou, 2006).

In summary, we know that high-protein diets increase calcium excretion but the effect of high-protein diets on calcium absorption is still unclear. High acid-forming diets tend to increase calcium excretion, whereas a more alkaline-forming diet (rich in fruit and vegetables) decreases calcium excretion. Therefore, if you eat a high-protein diet but do not have sufficient calcium, it stands to reason that, over time, you may lose calcium from your bones. You may be able to limit this loss by increasing the amount of alkaline-forming foods (fruit and vegetables) in the diet and limiting, or eliminating all animal protein. Furthermore, research suggests that physical (especially weight-bearing) exercise is the most critical factor for maintaining healthy bones, followed by improving diet and lifestyle; this means eating plenty of fresh fruit and vegetables, and cutting down on caffeine and avoiding alcohol and smoking.

For more information see Viva!Health's fully-referenced scientific report *Break Free – How to Build Healthy Bones and What Really Matters in the Prevention of Osteoporosis* and easy-to-read guide *Building Bones for Life* at: www.vegetarian.org.uk/campaigns/bones.

Conclusion

The realisation is growing that changing our diet can have an enormous impact on health – for better or worse. But what constitutes healthy food – and unhealthy – is not universally agreed and seems to change on a weekly basis. Cow's milk is vigorously defended by the dairy industry and they have managed to turn it into a national icon. Woe-betide anyone who challenges their sacred cow. Not surprisingly, the resulting controversy is confusing. On the one hand consumers are told that milk is essential for good bone health while on the other, that it causes allergies, illness and disease.

Of course we need calcium for bones and teeth as well as blood clotting, muscle function and regulating the heart's rhythm. But no matter how loudly the dairy industry shouts, an increasing body of evidence begs the question: is cow's milk really the best source of calcium? It certainly is not for most of the world's people. Claims that dairy is best carry strong overtones of cultural imperialism and simply ignore the 70 per cent of the global population who obtain their calcium from other sources – people such as the Japanese who traditionally have consumed no dairy yet have far better health than British people and live considerably longer.

Milk has been part of the human diet for less than 8,000 years – this is very recent in evolutionary terms. It is not just that most people don't drink it –

they cannot because their bodies will not tolerate it. Up to 100 per cent of some ethnic groups are lactose intolerant. It's obvious that the claims made for milk ignore the research and owe more to marketing hype than science.

The dairy industry has spent many years and many millions promoting the notion that cow's milk is good for us through expensive advertising campaigns such as the 'White Stuff' – fronted by the milk-moustachioed celebrity, Nell McAndrew. Now, because of an increasing body of evidence, there are signs of a growing realisation that milk is neither natural nor healthy.

The very people who are most aggressively targeted by the dairy industry – the young – are those most at risk of being damaged by milk. It is not just the few per cent under the age of one who will develop allergies but those likely to develop type 1 diabetes from cow's milk infant formula. The evidence is convincing even though the mechanism may not yet be fully understood. This is not the time to be withdrawing support from the midwives and infant feeding coordinators, who encourage breastfeeding in parts of the country with the lowest uptake.

Author of the world-famous book, *Baby and Child Care*, Dr Benjamin Spock, withdrew his support for cow's milk in 1998. In 1999, a study published in the

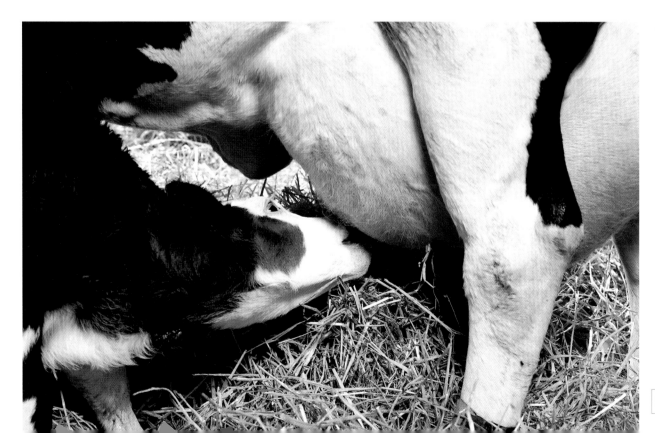

Journal of Pediatric Surgery reported that gastrointestinal bleeding caused by an allergic response to milk was a major cause of rectal bleeding in infancy, leading to iron-deficiency anaemia. This is now universally accepted. The World Health Organisation recommends that infants should be exclusively breastfed for the first six months of life in preference to being given cow's milk or soya formulas.

But it's not all about infants; cow's milk was linked to teenage acne in a study published in the *Journal of the American Academy of Dermatology*. In the same year, the journal Pediatrics published a review article concluding that there is scant evidence that consuming more milk and dairy products promotes better bone health in either children or adolescents. Since then, more evidence has built on these findings.

T. Colin Campbell, professor emeritus of nutritional biochemistry at Cornell University, culminated a lifetime of research with *The China Study*, one of the most comprehensive nutritional studies ever undertaken. Campbell agrees there is little evidence to show that increasing calcium intake will prevent fractures. In fact, research is moving in the opposite direction, showing that the more dairy and animal protein that is consumed, the higher the incidence of osteoporosis.

Cow's milk is clearly implicated in disease in both the young and old. Both UK arthritis charities, Arthritis Care and the Arthritis Research UK, agree that moving away from fatty foods such as meat and dairy and towards a diet rich in fruit, vegetables, and whole grains can help people with arthritis.

The rate at which some cancers are increasing is also a matter of concern. When Professor Jane Plant wrote *Your Life in Your Hands*, an account of how she overcame breast cancer by eliminating dairy, one in 10 UK women were affected by the disease. That was in 2000. When this report was first written in 2006, the figure had gone up to one in nine women. Now in 2014, a shocking one in eight women will develop breast cancer at some point in their lives!

Female breast cancer incidence rates in Britain have increased by almost 70 per cent since the mid-1970s. Just in the last ten years they have gone up by six per cent. In rural China, on the other hand, where very little if any dairy is consumed, just one in 10,000 women gets breast cancer. These figures should be shouted from the rooftops as a basis for action. Plant and Campbell – and many others for that matter – are in no doubt that cow's milk and dairy foods are responsible.

A point that is consistently overlooked is that two-thirds of the UK's milk comes from pregnant cows and as every mum knows, hormone levels during pregnancy can rise dramatically. This is no laughing matter as prostate, ovarian and colorectal cancer are all implicated. These cancers and the so-called diseases of affluence, such as diabetes, obesity, heart disease and even osteoporosis, occur increasingly in the countries that consume the most dairy products. It is not rocket science… cow's milk and dairy products cause disease.

The conclusions of this report are drawn from a huge body of peer-reviewed research from academic institutions all around the world. While the majority was done in an academic environment involving clinical trials or statistical analysis, some is of a more personal nature. Professor Jane Plant's spirit and courage in overcoming breast cancer through the elimination of all dairy could not fail to inspire the increasing number of women who are affected by this type of cancer.

Plant did not set out to promote one type of diet above another but as a scientist (geochemist) she took an analytical approach to the problem of cancer and ultimately found the solution: a dairy-free diet. Similarly, what initiated Campbell's extensive China study was not an attempt to justify or promote vegetarianism. In fact, Campbell grew up on a farm in northern Virginia and for much of his life ate the typical North American diet high in meat, eggs, whole milk and butter. He began his academic life trying to increase animal protein production. It was evidence from his own laboratory research that pointed an accusing finger at animal protein as a trigger for many diseases and he set out to confirm it through epidemiological research. For health reasons, he and his family now eat a vegan diet.

The World Health Organisation believes that the only way people can improve their health is through informed opinion and their own, active co-operation. We agree! As a science-based health charity, Viva!Health provides unbiased information on which people can make informed choices. We monitor and interpret scientific research on diet and health and communicate those findings to the public, health professionals, schools and food manufacturers. Importantly, we have no commercial or vested interests and offer a vital – and what sometimes feels like a solitary – source of accurate and unbiased information.

This report combines the findings of over 400

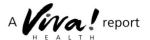

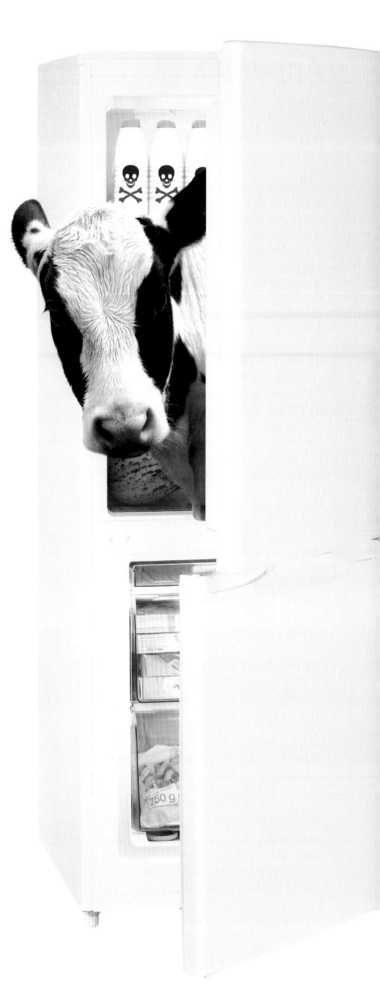

scientific papers from reputable peer-reviewed journals such as the *British Medical Journal* and the *Lancet*. The research is clear – the consumption of cow's milk and dairy products is linked to the development of teenage acne, allergies, arthritis, some cancers, colic, constipation, coronary heart disease, Crohn's disease, diabetes, dementia, ear infection, food poisoning, gallstones, kidney disease, migraine, autoimmune conditions, including multiple sclerosis, overweight, obesity and osteoporosis.

As a species, we do not need saturated animal fat, animal protein or cholesterol. We do not need the trans fatty acids in processed foods. We do not need salt and sugar in their current quantities. We do need to move towards a plant-based, whole grain diet containing a wide range of fruits, vegetables, grains, pulses, nuts and seeds for the nutrients that will promote a long and healthy life.

These, of course, are the same foods which contain protection against disease in the form of antioxidants and fibre. What is killing the Western world are the degenerative diseases associated with affluence. It is clear that the same diet that is good for preventing cancer is also good for preventing heart disease, obesity, diabetes and so on.

The official approach to the causes of all these diseases remains extremely equivocal and dietary advice seems to be based far more on not upsetting particular vested interests than improving the public's health. As a consequence, no matter how much money is thrown at the NHS, the incidence of all these diseases goes on increasing remorselessly because public health policy is geared almost exclusively towards cure rather than prevention. It is predicted that by 2020 almost one in two people (47 per cent) will get cancer in their lifetime and that by 2035 the NHS will be spending 17 per cent of its entire budget on treating diabetes alone. This is clearly unsustainable and we need to start looking for preventative measures.

Only when prevention assumes the pre-eminence it should have will the avoidance of dairy and other animal products be seen as central to improving public health. Meanwhile, it is left to individuals to discover what they can about diet and heath while Government health policy continues to kill us and sows the seeds for the destruction of our own children's health, most of which will germinate in early adulthood. It is a national disgrace and an evolutionary disaster.

Appendix I
The Safety of Soya

Soya milk, made from soya beans, contains the same amount of protein as dairy milk. It also provides all eight of the essential amino acids which the human body requires. Soya milk is rich in polyunsaturated fatty acids including omega-3, and is free of cholesterol. Compared to cow's milk, soya milk contains lower levels of saturated fat and higher levels of unsaturated essential fatty acids which can lower cholesterol levels in the body. Soya products provide an excellent source of B vitamins, calcium, iron and zinc. Soya also contains fibre which is important for good bowel health and can also lower cholesterol.

In recent years, soya milk and soya-based products have received much attention because of the phytoestrogens that they contain. Phytoestrogens are plant-made substances that can act in a similar way to the hormone oestrogen, although they are far less potent (Coldham et al., 1997). They are found in many fruits, vegetables, dried beans, peas, and whole grains. Isoflavones are a type of phytoestrogen found in soya beans and include genistein and daidzein. In general, much of the data indicates that isoflavones are beneficial to health. For example, isoflavones may have a protective role against heart disease. Extensive research has shown that soya protein can lower blood cholesterol levels. The American Food and Drug Administration and the UK Joint Health Claim Initiative approved following health claim: the inclusion of at least 25g of soya protein per day, as part of a diet low in saturated fat, can help reduce blood cholesterol levels (FDA, 1999; JHCI, 2002). In a recent review of soya research it was reported that soya protein could lower LDL ('bad') cholesterol by 3-5 per cent, which is similar to the effects of soluble fibre. The author if this review says that even this modest reduction is meaningful, because in theory, over time, each one per cent decrease in LDL cholesterol reduces heart disease risk and/or mortality by as much as 2-5 per cent (Messina, 2010).

In addition to the benefits to heart health, isoflavones have been shown to offer other health benefits. For example, they may have a role in reducing menopausal symptoms; dietary soya supplementation has been shown to substantially reduce the frequency of hot flushes in some postmenopausal women (Albertazzi et al, 1998). While only a few clinical studies have examined the influence of phytoestrogens on bone health, a review of the current research states that the collective data suggests that diets rich in phytoestrogens have bone-sparing effects in the long term, in other words the data indicates that phytoestrogens may be beneficial to bone health (Setchell and Lydeking-Olsen, 2003).

Conversely, research focusing on the hormonal content of cow's milk has not been widely discussed and surprisingly very little research has been published on this topic. Cow's milk contains the hormones oestrogen, progesterone and a range of hormone precursors (androstenedione, dehydroepiandrosterone-sulphate, and 5 -reduced steroids like 5 -androstanedione, 5 -pregnanedione, and dihydrotestosterone). Some researchers are particularly concerned about the oestrogen content of cow's milk (Ganmaa and Sato, 2005), suggesting that cow's milk is one of the important routes of human exposure to oestrogens. What concerns them is that the nature of cow's milk has changed drastically over the last hundred years, in that for most of the time that a cow is milked, she is also pregnant and therefore secreting hormones into the milk. The levels of these hormones in cow's milk increases markedly during pregnancy and has been linked to a wide range of illnesses and diseases including certain hormone-dependent cancers such as ovarian and breast cancer.

Consistent levels of soya isoflavones have been a component of the diet of many populations for centuries and the consumption of soya is generally regarded as beneficial for health with a potentially protective effect against a number of chronic diseases because of their oestrogenic activity. A 2003 review concluded that when viewed in its entirety, the literature supports the safety of isoflavones as typically consumed in diets based on soya or containing soya products (Munro et al., 2003). More recently, a review of 20 years of soya research concluded that, other than allergic reactions, there is almost no credible evidence to suggest traditional soya foods exert clinically relevant adverse effects in healthy individuals when consumed in amounts consistent with Asian intake (Messina, 2010).

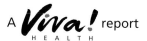
Soya-based Infant Formula

Because soya-based infant formula is such a popular alternative to cow's milk formula, it was decided to include a separate section on it here. Soya protein-based nutrition during infancy has a long history of safe use around the world dating back centuries. The first report of soya-based infant formula in the West was recorded in 1909 (Ruhrah, 1909) and soya-based infant formula was used in cases of infantile eczema as early as in the 1920s (Hill and Stuart, 1929). Since these early days soya-based infant formula has come a long way; it now contains all the nutrients needed by an infant and can be used as a safe alternative or supplement to breast milk if necessary.

Soya-based infant formulas have been widely used since the 1960s. In the US, the prevalence of feeding with soya-based infant formula can be as high as 36 per cent (Merritt and Jenks, 2004). In contrast, in most European countries, feeding with soya-based infant formula is largely restricted to infants who are allergic to or intolerant of cow's milk formula. The prevalence of soya-based infant formula feeding in the UK tends to be less than two per cent (COT, 2003). In 2000, a survey conducted on behalf of the Department of Health, the Scottish Executive, the National Assembly for Wales and the Department of Health, Social Services and Public Safety in Northern Ireland reported that soya formula was fed to approximately one per cent of non-breastfed infants aged four to 10 weeks rising to approximately two per cent of infants aged 10-14 weeks (Hamlyn et al., 2002).

The UK government currently advises that you shouldn't give your baby soya-based infant formula unless your GP or health visitor advises you to (NHS Choices, 2013g). They also state that in almost all cases, breastfeeding or another type of formula will be a better choice, and suggest that if you are giving your baby soya-based infant formula at the moment, you should talk to your GP or health visitor about changing to a different formula. This reflects concerns about the use of soya-based infant formulas. Based largely on anecdotal and animal-based experimental evidence, these concerns have focused on the nutritional adequacy of soya-based infant formula, the effect of phytoestrogens, genetically modified soya and the effects of glucose syrup (which is used in place of lactose). These concerns are addressed below.

Nutritional adequacy

Soya-based infant formulas are formulated to meet all of the nutrient requirements of the growing infant. A number of studies have documented normal growth and development in infants fed soya-based infant formulas. One study compared weight, length and head circumference of healthy term infants to one year of age, fed either soya-based formula, or exclusively breastfed for at least two months then weaned on to cow's milk formula. Results demonstrated similar growth in the first year of life between groups (Lasekan et al., 1999). Another, more recent study compared the nutritional status and growth of 168 infants who were allergic to cow's milk and were fed either soya-based infant formula or extensively hydrolysed whey formula. Results showed that in both groups, nutrient intake and growth were within reference values confirming the safety and effectiveness of the soya-based formula (Seppo et al., 2005). Current evidence indicates that soya-based infant formulas ensure normal growth and development in healthy term infants (Turck, 2007).

Unfortunately there is currently no infant formula available in the UK which is suitable for vegans since Heinz discontinued their Nurture Soya (formerly Farley's Soya Formula) in 2010. There are soya formulas available (such as SMA's Wysoy and Cow and Gate's Infasoy), but these are not suitable for vegans as they are fortified with vitamin D3, which is made from lanolin (a soft waxy substance secreted by the sebaceous glands of sheep).

Phytoestrogens

The role of phytoestrogens in the diet has become a somewhat controversial area with warnings focusing particularly on the safety of soya-based infant formulas. Various animal experiments (primarily using rodents and primates) have suggested that phytoestrogens can elicit oestrogenic effects with respect to sexual development and reproductive function. However, it is widely acknowledged that the results of animal experiments should not form the basis of a public health policy as significant differences in biological function between rodents, primates and humans make the interpretation of these types of experimental studies extremely difficult. Just one single human study has specifically examined the effect of soya formula feeding on sexual development and fertility (Strom et al., 2001). This study examined the association between exposure to soya formula in infancy and reproductive health in adulthood. The results provided no evidence of adverse clinical effects on sexual development or reproductive health of males and females. Indeed the authors of this study stated that their findings were reassuring about the safety of infant soya formula.

In 1998, a review on isoflavones, soya-based infant formulas and hormone function reported that growth was normal and no changes in timing of puberty or in infertility rates were reported in humans who consumed soya formulas as infants (Klein, 1998). The author concluded that soya-based infant formulas continue to be a safe, nutritionally complete feeding option for most infants.

However in 2003, in response to concerns about the oestrogenic properties of phytoestrogens the UK Department of Health's committee of independent experts, the Committee on Toxicity of Chemicals in Food, Consumer Products and the Environment (COT) reviewed the health aspects of phytoestrogens as part of an ongoing programme of reviews on naturally-occurring chemicals (COT, 2003). This report attempted to assess, on the basis of current evidence, if ingestion of soya-based infant formulas poses any risk for human infants.

The report compared estimated dietary isoflavone intakes in Western and Eastern populations and found that Eastern populations have a significantly higher intake of phytoestrogens. While in the UK, the US, Australia and New Zealand isoflavone intakes tended to range from around 0.8 milligrams per day to 17.0 milligrams per day, intakes in Japan, China and Korea ranged from 18.0 milligrams per day to 200 milligrams per day. These figures did not include data collected from one group of vegans in New Zealand whose intake was found to be 140.0 milligrams per day (COT, 2003). The COT estimated that the daily isoflavone intake of a soya formula fed infant was approximately 40 milligrams per day (COT, 2003), above the average Western intake but well within the range of intakes seen in Eastern countries.

In a cautionary statement the COT warned that isoflavones may lower free thyroxine concentrations and advised that physicians and other health care workers be aware of possible interactions between isoflavones in soya-based infant formulas and thyroid function, particularly in infants with congenital hypothyroidism. That said, the report concluded that the findings from a wide range of studies did not provide direct evidence that phytoestrogens present in soya-based infant formulas can adversely affect

the health of infants. However, they said that the findings did provide evidence of potential risks. For this reason, the Scientific Advisory Committee on Nutrition (SACN) considered there to be no substantive medical need for, nor health benefit arising from, the use of soya-based infant formulas and together with the COT recommended that the Department of Health reviewed current advice on the use of soya-based infant formulas.

The report did acknowledge that there is no evidence that populations which habitually ingest high quantities of soya (such as the Chinese or Japanese) have impaired fertility or altered sexual development. Despite this, they recommended that research should be undertaken as a matter of high priority to determine whether ingestion of soya-based formulas can affect infant reproductive development in any way. Interestingly, the United Kingdom and New Zealand are the only countries to have issued such advice with specific reference to phytoestrogens and soya-based infant formulas.

This is a controversial issue which has yet to be resolved. The FSA advise that, until a full review of the evidence both supporting and opposing soya formula has been completed, there is no reason to stop your baby having a soya formula if it has been suggested by a health professional. This it would seem is erring of the side of extreme caution given that thousands of babies have been raised on soya-based infant formula.

Genetically modified soya
It is relatively recently that the genetic modification (GM) of organisms (plants and animals) has developed as a technology. However, GM technology has not been welcomed by the British public; many people are deeply suspicious and mistrustful of the science. We have been reassured in the past that certain foods are quite safe to eat only to find that they are not. Many of us will remember in 1990, just before the bovine spongiform encephalopathy (BSE) crisis, John Gummer feeding his daughter a beef burger and saying that beef was perfectly safe, it was not.

The mistrust remains and many questions have gone unanswered. For example, have the transgenic plants grown so far met expectations? Evidence suggests that in many cases they have not met the high yields expected. What is the real risk of transgenic contamination between genetically modified (GM) and unmodified plants? This question refers to the contamination of an unmodified crop with pollen from a GM plant. The pollen of the GM plant will carry copies of the foreign genes that were used confer some additional characteristic to the plant. These may encode pesticide resistance for example along with antibiotic resistance marker genes that were used to identify the successfully modified plants when they were first produced. The question of contamination is difficult to answer as it may be years or even decades before we can assess the full extent of transgenic contamination, but so far evidence suggests widespread contamination has occurred in some parts of the world.

Another concern is that the genetic material (DNA or genes) may be transferred from GM foods to bacteria in the human gut and from there into human tissue. There is experimental evidence that DNA from GM soya has been taken up by bacteria in the small intestines of human volunteers (Netherwood et al., 2004). This raises concerns that bacteria in the gut (for example Lactobacillus) might then transfer that DNA into our intestinal epithelial cells. What effect this may have on human health will largely depend on what the gene does; it may do nothing but is that a risk worth taking? Finally, as a result of a lack of funding, scientists are sometimes forced to adopt the corporate agenda, which is not necessarily the same as the public good. For example, Monsanto has used genetic engineering to produce herbicide resistance crops thus increasing sales of its herbicide Roundup.

GM products, especially soya and maize, are now in so many foods, including baby milks, that it can be difficult to avoid them. We do not yet know enough about this technology to confidently say what the long term effects of it will be but consumers appear to be voting with their shopping baskets by avoiding GM foods as far as possible. SMA Nutrition and Cow and Gate state that no GM soya is used in their soya-based infant formulas (SMA Careline, 2014; Cow and Gate, 2014).

Glucose syrup and tooth decay

Another concern with infant soya formula is that the glucose syrup content may harm teeth. All infant formulas must comply with standards laid down by UK regulations which specify minimum and maximum amounts of carbohydrate (the body's main form of energy). The carbohydrate in cow's milk is the sugar lactose, in soya-based infant formula an alternative carbohydrate is used: glucose syrup. Glucose syrup is often confused with sugars but in fact is derived from corn starch and is not the same

as glucose or syrup. It is mainly made up of beneficial complex carbohydrates (starches) rather than simple carbohydrates (sugars) which are known to be harmful to teeth. Research has shown that soya infant formulas are no more likely to cause tooth decay than other infant formulas (Moynihan, 1996).

Tooth decay can be the result of many factors, not only the presence of sugars in a food and drink but how they are consumed. It has been shown that prolonged contact of sugary foods and drinks with teeth increases the risk of tooth decay significantly. Children should be encouraged to drink water if they are thirsty as it quenches the thirst, maintains body fluid levels, does not spoil the appetite and is safe for teeth. Fresh fruit juice provides a good source of vitamin C and can be given with meals to help the absorption of iron. However, fresh fruit juices are acidic so may be harmful to teeth and should be diluted with water. Furthermore, juice should be served in a cup rather than a bottle to minimise the risk of tooth decay. Children should be discouraged from consuming sugary carbonated drinks and squashes as these contribute to dental problems, are a poor source of nutrients and tend to displace other more nutritious foods. If normal weaning practices are adopted, soya infant formulas should not cause harm to teeth (Moynihan, 1996).

In summary, soya-based infant formulas continue to provide a safe feeding option for most infants. They meet all the nutritional requirements of the infant with none of the detrimental effects associated with the consumption of cow's milk formulas.

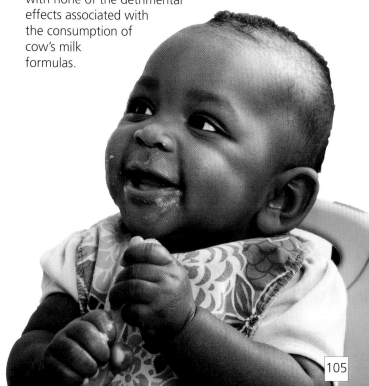

Appendix II
Body Mass Index

Table 1. Body mass index (BMI) table in imperial units. Find the nearest height in feet and inches on the top row. Read down that column to find the nearest weight in stones and pounds. Then find your BMI in the left hand column.

BMI	4FT10IN	4FT11IN	5FT 0IN	5FT 1IN	5FT 2IN	5FT 3IN	5FT 4IN
17.0	5st11lb	6st0lb	6st3lb	6st5lb	6st8lb	6st11lb	7st1lb
18.5	6st4lb	6st7lb	6st10lb	6st13lb	7st3lb	7st6lb	7st9lb
20.0	6st11lb	7st1lb	7st4lb	7st7lb	7st11lb	8st0lb	8st4lb
22.5	7st9lb	7st13b	8st3lb	8st7lb	8st11lb	9st1lb	9st5lb
25.0	8st7lb	8st11lb	9st2lb	9st6lb	9st10lb	10st1lb	10st5lb
27.5	9st5lb	9st10lb	10st0lb	10st5lb	10lb10lb	11st1lb	11st6lb
30.0	10st3lb	10st8lb	10st13lb	11st4lb	11st10lb	12st1lb	12st6lb
32.5	11st1lb	11st6lb	11st12lb	12st4lb	12st9lb	13st1lb	13st7lb
35.0	11st13lb	12st5lb	12st11lb	13st3lb	13st9lb	14st1lb	14st7lb

BMI	5FT 5IN	5FT 6IN	5FT 7IN	5FT 8IN	5FT 9IN	5FT10IN	5FT11IN
17.0	7st4lb	7st7lb	7st10lb	7st13lb	8st3lb	8st6lb	8st9lb
18.5	7st13lb	8st2lb	8st6lb	8st9lb	8st13lb	9st2lb	9st6lb
20.0	8st8lb	8st11lb	9st1lb	9st5lb	9st9lb	9st13lb	10st3lb
22.5	9st9lb	9st13lb	10st3lb	10st7lb	10st12lb	11st2lb	11st7lb
25.0	10st10lb	11st0lb	11st5lb	11st10lb	12st1lb	12st6lb	12st11lb
27.5	11st11lb	12st2lb	12st7lb	12st12lb	13st4lb	13st0lb	14st1lb
30.0	12st12lb	13st3lb	13st9lb	14st1lb	14st7lb	14st13lb	15st5lb
32.5	13st13lb	14st5lb	14st11lb	15st3lb	15st10lb	16st2lb	16st9lb
35.0	15st0lb	15st6lb	15st13lb	16st6lb	16st13lb	17st5lb	17st12lb

BMI	6FT 0IN	6FT 1IN	6FT 2IN	6FT 3IN	6FT 4IN	6FT 5IN	
17.0	8st13lb	9st2lb	9st6lb	9st10lb	9st13lb	10st3lb	
18.5	9st10lb	10st0lb	10st4lb	10st8lb	10st11lb	11st2lb	
20.0	10st7lb	10st11lb	11st1lb	11st6lb	11st10lb	12st0lb	
22.5	11st11lb	12st2lb	12st7lb	12st12lb	13st2lb	13st7lb	
25.0	13st2lb	13st7lb	13st12lb	14st4lb	14st9lb	15st0lb	
27.5	14st6lb	14st12lb	15st4lb	15st10lb	16st1lb	16st7lb	
30.0	15st11lb	16st3lb	16st9lb	17st2lb	17st8lb	18st1lb	
32.5	17st1lb	17st8lb	18st1lb	18st8lb	19st1lb	19st8lb	
35.0	18st6lb	18st13lb	19st6lb	20st0lb	20st7lb	21st8lb	

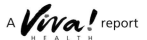

References

Abelow BJ, Holford TR, and Insogna KL. 1992. Cross-cultural association between dietary animal protein and hip fracture: a hypothesis. *Calcified Tissue International*. 50 (1) 14-18.

Adebamowo CA, Spiegelman D, Danby FW, Frazier AL, Willett WC and Holmes MD. 2005. High school dietary dairy intake and teenage acne. *Journal of the American Academy of Dermatology*. 52 (2) 207-214.

Adebamowo CA, Spiegelman D, Berkey CS, Danby FW, Rockett HH, Colditz GA, Willett WC and Holmes MD. 2006. Milk consumption and acne in adolescent girls. *Dermatology Online Journal*. 12 (4) 1.

Adebamowo CA, Spiegelman D, Berkey CS, Danby FW, Rockett HH, Colditz GA, Willett WC and Holmes MD. 2008. Milk consumption and acne in teenaged boys. *Journal of the American Academy of Dermatology*. 58 (5) 787-793.

AbuGhazaleh AA, Schingoethe DJ, Hippen AR, and Kalscheur KF. 2004. Conjugated linoleic acid increases in milk when cows fed fish meal and extruded soybeans for an extended period of time. *Journal of Dairy Science*. 87 (6) 1758-1766.

Agranoff BW and Goldberg D. 1974. Diet and the geographical distribution of multiple sclerosis. *The Lancet*. 2 (7888) 1061-1066.

Adlercreutz H. 1990. Western diet and Western diseases: some hormonal and biochemical mechanisms and associations. *Scandinavian Journal of Clinical Laboratory Investigation Supplementum*. 201, 3-23.

Albertazzi, P., Pansini, F., Bonaccorsi, G., Zanotti, L., Forini, E. and De Aloysio, D. 1998. The effect of dietary soy supplementation on hot flushes. *Obstetrics and Gynecology*. 91 (1) 6-11.

Alexy U, Remer T, Manz F, Neu CM and Schoenau E. 2005. Long-term protein intake and dietary potential renal acid load are associated with bone modeling and remodeling at the proximal radius in healthy children. *American Journal of Clinical Nutrition*. 82 (5) 1107-1114.

Allen NE, Appleby PN, Davey GK and Key TJ. 2000. Hormones and diet: low insulin-like growth factor-I but normal bioavailable androgens in vegan men. *British Journal of Cancer*. 83 (1) 95-97.

Allen NE, Key TJ, Appleby PN, Travis RC, Roddam AW, Rinaldi S, Egevad L, Rohrmann S, Linseisen J, Pischon T, Boeing H, Johnsen NF, Tjønneland A, Grønbaek H, Overvad K, Kiemeney L, Bueno-de-Mesquita HB, Bingham S, Khaw KT, Tumino R, Berrino F, Mattiello A, Sacerdote C, Palli D, Quirós JR, Ardanaz E, Navarro C, Larrañaga N, Gonzalez C, Sanchez MJ, Trichopoulou A, Travezea C, Trichopoulos D, Jenab M, Ferrari P, Riboli E and Kaaks R. 2007. Serum insulin-like growth factor (IGF)-I and IGF-binding protein-3 concentrations and prostate cancer risk: results from the European Prospective Investigation into Cancer and Nutrition. *Cancer Epidemiology Biomarkers and Prevention*. 16 (6) 1121-1127.

Allen NE, Key TJ, Appleby PN, Travis RC, Roddam AW, Tjønneland A, Johnsen NF, Overvad K, Linseisen J, Rohrmann S, Boeing H, Pischon T, Bueno-de-Mesquita HB, Kiemeney L, Tagliabue G, Palli D, Vineis P, Tumino R, Trichopoulou A, Kassapa C, Trichopoulos D, Ardanaz E, Larrañaga N, Tormo MJ, González CA, Quirós JR, Sánchez MJ, Bingham S, Khaw KT, Manjer J, Berglund G, Stattin P, Hallmans G, Slimani N, Ferrari P, Rinaldi S and Riboli E. 2008. Animal foods, protein, calcium and prostate cancer risk: the European Prospective Investigation into Cancer and Nutrition. *British Journal of Cancer*. 98 (9) 1574-1581.

Allergy UK, 2005. *Migraine*. (Fact sheet) London: Allergy UK.

Allergy UK, 2012. *Hay Fever and Allergic Rhinitis* [online]. Available from: www.allergyuk.org/hayfever-and-allergic-rhinitis/hay-fever-and-allergic-rhinitis [Accessed 17 September 2013].

American Academy of Pediatrics, Committee on Nutrition. 1992. The use of whole cows' milk in infancy. *Pediatrics*. 89, 1105-1109.

Anderson JW, Johnstone BM and Remley DT. 1999. Breast-feeding and cognitive development: a meta-analysis. *American Journal of Clinical Nutrition*. 70 (4) 525-535.

Anderson JW. 1986. Dietary fiber in nutrition management of diabetes. In: G. Vahouny, V. and D. Kritchevsky (eds.), *Dietary fiber: Basic and Clinical Aspects*. New York: Plenum Press.

Anderson JW, Smith BM and Geil PB. 1990. High-fiber diet for diabetes. Safe and effective treatment. *Postgraduate Medicine*. 88 (2) 157-161, 164, 167-168.

Anderson JW, Randles KM, Kendall CW and Jenkins DJ. 2004. Carbohydrate and fiber recommendations for individuals with diabetes: a quantitative assessment and meta-analysis of the evidence. *Journal of the American College of Nutrition*. 23 (1) 5-17.

Andiran F, Dayi S, and Mete E. 2003. Cow's milk consumption in constipation and anal fissure in infants and young children. *Journal of Paediatrics and Child Health*. 39 (5) 329-331.

Appleby PN, Thorogood M, Mann JI and Key TJ. 1999. The Oxford Vegetarian Study: an overview. *American Journal of Clinical Nutrition*. 70 (3 Suppl) 525S-531S.

Appleby P, Roddam A, Allen N, Key T. 2007. Comparative fracture risk in vegetarians and nonvegetarians in EPIC-Oxford. *European Journal of Clinical Nutrition*. 61 (12) 1400-1406.

Arenz S, Rückerl R, Koletzko B and von Kries R. (2004) Breastfeeding and Childhood obesity: a systematic review. *International Journal of Obesity Related Metabolic Disorders*. 28: 1247-1256.

Arthritis Research UK, 2013. *Who gets arthritis?* [online]. Available from: www.arthritisresearchuk.org/arthritis-information/conditions/arthritis/who-gets-it.aspx [Accessed 17 September 2013].

Arthritis Research UK, 2013a. *Do vegetarian or vegan diets help?* [online]. Available from: www.arthritisresearchuk.org/arthritis-information/arthritis-and-daily-life/diet-and-arthritis/do-vegetarian-or-vegan-diets-help.aspx [Accessed 17 September 2013].

Arthritis Research UK, 2013b. *Who Foods and supplements that might help* [online]. Available from: www.arthritisresearchuk.org/arthritis-information/arthritis-and-daily-life/diet-and-arthritis/foods-and-supplements-that-might-help.aspx [Accessed 17 September 2013].

Arthritis Care, 2010. *Calcium Fact Sheet* [online] Available from: www.arthritiscare.org.uk/PublicationsandResources/Listedbytype/Factsheets/main_content/CalciumFactsheetMay10.pdf [Accessed 17 September 2013].

Arthritis Care, 2011. *Eating well* [online] Available from: www.arthritiscare.org.uk/LivingwithArthritis/Self-management/Eatingwell [Accessed 17 September 2013].

Ashwell M, Stone E, Mathers J, Barnes S, Compston J, Francis RM, Key T, Cashman KD, Cooper C, Khaw KT, Lanham-New S, Macdonald H, Prentice A, Shearer M and Stephen A. 2008. Nutrition and bone health projects funded by the UK Food Standards Agency: have they helped to inform public health policy? *British Journal of Nutrition*. 99 (1) 198-205.

Atkins PJ. 2005. Fattening Children or Fattening Farmers? School Milk in Britain, 1921-1941. *Economic History Review*. 58 (1) 57-78.

Aune D, Lau R, Chan DS, Vieira R, Greenwood DC, Kampman E and Norat T. 2012. Dairy products and colorectal cancer risk: a systematic review and meta-analysis of cohort studies. *Annals of Oncology*. 23 (1) 37-45.

Autschbach F, Eisold S, Hinz U, Zinser S, Linnebacher M, Giese T, Loffler T, Buchler MW and Schmidt J. 2005. High prevalence of Mycobacterium avium subspecies paratuberculosis IS900 DNA in gut tissues from individuals with Crohn's disease. *Gut*. 54 (7) 944-949.

Axelsson I, Gebre-Medhin M, Hernell O, Jakobsonn I, Michaelsen KF and Samuelson G. 1999. Recommendations for prevention of iron deficiency. Delay cow's milk intake as a beverage to infants until 10-12 months of age. *Läkartidningen*. 96, 2206-2208.

Aydogan B, Kiroglu M, Altintas D, Yilmaz M, Yorgancilar E and Tuncer U. 2004. The role of food allergy in otitis media with effusion. *Otolaryngology and Head and Neck Surgery*. 130 (6) 747-750.

Bajekal M, Scholes S, Love H, Hawkins N, O'Flaherty M, Raine R and Capewell S. 2012. Analysing recent socioeconomic trends in coronary heart disease mortality in England, 2000-2007: a population modelling study. *PLoS Medicine*. 9 (6) e1001237.

Baker JR. 1990. Grey seal (Halichoerus grypus) milk composition and its variation over lactation. *The British Veterinary Journal*, 146 (3) 233-238.

Ballard O and Morrow AL. 2013. Human milk composition: nutrients and bioactive factors. *Pediatric Clinics of North America*. 60 (1) 49-74.

Barnard N. 1998. *Foods that fight pain*. New York, US: Three Rivers Press.

Barnard ND, Scialli AR, Turner-McGrievy G, Lanou AJ and Glass J. 2005. The effects of a low-fat, plant-based dietary intervention on body weight, metabolism, and insulin sensitivity. *The American Journal of Medicine*. 118 (9) 991-997.

Barnard ND, Cohen J, Jenkins DJ, Turner-McGrievy G, Gloede L, Green A and Ferdowsian H. 2009. A low-fat vegan diet and a conventional diabetes diet in the treatment of type 2 diabetes: a randomized, controlled, 74-wk clinical trial. *American Journal of Clinical Nutrition*. 89 (5) 1588S-1596S.

Barnard ND, Katcher HI, Jenkins DJ, Cohen J and Turner-McGrievy G. Vegetarian and vegan diets in type 2 diabetes management. 2009a. *Nutrition Reviews*. 67 (5) 255-263.

Barr SI. 2003. Increased dairy product or calcium intake: is body weight or composition affected in humans? *Journal of Nutrition*. 133 (1) 245S-248S.

Barreiro C, Albano H, Silva J and Teixeira P. 2013. Role of flies as vectors of foodborne pathogens in rural areas. ISRN *Microbiology*. 2013:718780.

Barzel US and Jowsey J. 1969. The effects of chronic acid and alkali administration on bone turnover. *Clinical Science*. 36. 517-524.

Bates B, Lennox A and Swan G. 2010. *NDNS Headline results from Year 1 of the Rolling Programme (2008/2009)* [online]. www.food.gov.uk/multimedia/pdfs/publication/ndnsreport0809.pdf [Accessed 23 October 2013].

Berkey CS, Rockett HR, Willett WC and Colditz GA. 2005. Milk, dairy fat, dietary calcium, and weight gain: a longitudinal study of adolescents. *Archives of Pediatric and Adolescent Medicine*. 159 (6) 543-550.

Berkow SE, Barnard ND, Saxe GA and Ankerberg-Nobis T. 2007. Diet and survival after prostate cancer diagnosis. *Nutrition Reviews*. 65 (9) 391-403.

Bernard JY, De Agostini M, Forhan A, Alfaiate T, Bonet M, Champion V, Kaminski M, de Lauzon-Guillain B, Charles MA and Heude B; EDEN Mother-Child Cohort Study Group. 2013. Breastfeeding duration and cognitive development at 2 and 3 years of age in the EDEN mother-child cohort. *Journal of Pediatrics*. 163 (1) 36-42.

Bernstein, J.M. 1993. The role of IgE-mediated hypersensitivity in the development of otitis media with effusion: a review. *Otolaryngology and Head and Neck Surgery*. 109 (3 Pt 2) 611-620.

Berry, E., Middleton, N., Gravenor, M. and Hillerton, E. 2003. *Science (or art) of cell counting. Proceedings of the British Mastitis Conference (2003) Garstang*. 73-83 [online]. Available from: www.britishmastitisconference.org.uk/BMC2003Proceedings.pdf [Accessed 9 September 2013].

BHF, 2012. British Heart Foundation. *Coronary heart disease statistics*. A compendium of health statistics [online] Available from: www.bhf.org.uk/publications/view-publication.aspx?ps=1002097 [Accessed 14 October 2013].

BHF, 2013. British Heart Foundation. *Cardiovascular disease statistics*. [online] Available from: www.bhf.org.uk/heart%20health/facts%20and%20statistics.aspx [Accessed 14 October 2013].

Bingham SA, Luben R, Welch A, Wareham N, Khaw KT and Day N. 2003. Are imprecise methods obscuring a relation between fat and breast cancer? *The Lancet*. 362 (9379) 212-214.

Bingham SA, Day NE, Luben R, Ferrari P, Slimani N, Norat T, Clavel-Chapelon F, Kesse E, Nieters A, Boeing H, Tjonneland A, Overvad K, Martinez C, Dorronsoro M, Gonzalez CA, Key TJ, Trichopoulou A, Naska A, Vineis P, Tumino R, Krogh V, Bueno-de-Mesquita HB, Peeters PH, Berglund G, Hallmans G, Lund E, Skeie G, Kaaks R and Riboli E; European Prospective Investigation into Cancer and Nutrition. 2003a. Dietary fibre in food and protection against colorectal cancer in the European Prospective Investigation into Cancer and Nutrition (EPIC): an observational study. *The Lancet*. 361 (9368) 1496-1501.

Bingham SA, Norat T, Moskal A, Ferrari P, Slimani N, Clavel-Chapelon F, Kesse E, Nieters A, Boeing H, Tjønneland A, Overvad K, Martinez C, Dorronsoro M, González CA, Ardanaz E, Navarro C, Quirós JR, Key TJ, Day NE, Trichopoulou A, Naska A, Krogh V, Tumino R, Palli D, Panico S, Vineis P, Bueno-de-Mesquita HB, Ocké MC, Peeters PH, Berglund G, Hallmans G, Lund E, Skeie G, Kaaks R and Riboli E. 2005. Is the association with fiber from foods in colorectal cancer confounded by folate intake? *Cancer Epidemiology Biomarkers and Prevention*. 14 (6) 1552-1556.

Bischoff-Ferrari HA, Dawson-Hughes B, Baron JA, Burckhardt P, Li R, Spiegelman D, Specker B, Orav JE, Wong JB, Staehelin HB, O'Reilly E, Kiel DP and Willett WC. 2007. Calcium intake and hip fracture risk in men and women: a meta-analysis of prospective cohort studies and randomized controlled trials. *American Journal of Clinical Nutrition*. 86 (6) 1780-1790.

Bischoff-Ferrari HA, Kiel DP, Dawson-Hughes B, Orav JE, Li R, Spiegelman D, Dietrich T and Willett WC. 2009. Dietary calcium and serum 25-hydroxyvitamin D status in relation to BMD among U.S. adults. *Journal of Bone and Mineral Research*. 24 (5) 935-942.

Blowey R and Edmondson P. 2000. *Mastitis Control in Dairy Herds*. UK: Farming Press Books.

BMA, 2013. British Medical Association. *Obesity, policy and facts* [online]. Available from: http://bma.org.uk/working-for-change/improving-and-protecting-health/obesity/obesity-policy-and-facts [Accessed 22 October 2013].

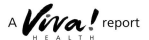

Boffetta P, Couto E, Wichmann J, Ferrari P, Trichopoulos D, Bueno-de-Mesquita HB, van Duijnhoven FJ, Büchner FL, Key T, Boeing H, Nöthlings U, Linseisen J, Gonzalez CA, Overvad K, Nielsen MR, Tjønneland A, Olsen A, Clavel-Chapelon F, Boutron-Ruault MC, Morois S, Lagiou P, Naska A, Benetou V, Kaaks R, Rohrmann S, Panico S, Sieri S, Vineis P, Palli D, van Gils CH, Peeters PH, Lund E, Brustad M, Engeset D, Huerta JM, Rodríguez L, Sánchez MJ, Dorronsoro M, Barricarte A, Hallmans G, Johansson I, Manjer J, Sonestedt E, Allen NE, Bingham S, Khaw KT, Slimani N, Jenab M, Mouw T, Norat T, Riboli E and Trichopoulou A. 2010. Fruit and vegetable intake and overall cancer risk in the European Prospective Investigation Into Cancer and Nutrition (EPIC). *Journal of the National Cancer Institute*. 102 (8) 529-537.

Bonjour JP. 2005. Dietary protein: an essential nutrient for bone health. *Journal of the American College of Nutrition*. 24. 526S-536S.

Boyd NF, Stone J, Vogt KN, Connelly BS, Martin LJ and Minkin S. 2003. Dietary fat and breast cancer risk revisited: a meta-analysis of the published literature. *British Journal of Cancer*. 89 (9) 1672-1685.

Breslau, N.A., Brinkley, L., Hill, K.D. and Pak C.Y. 1988. Relationship of animal protein-rich diet to kidney stone formation and calcium metabolism. *The Journal of Clinical Endocrinology and Metabolism*. 66 (1) 140-146.

Brown AC and Roy M. 2010 Does evidence exist to include dietary therapy in the treatment of Crohn's disease? *Expert Review of Gastroenterology and Hepatology*. 4 (2) 191-215.

Brown AC, Rampertab SD and Mullin GE. 2011 Existing dietary guidelines for Crohn's disease and ulcerative colitis. *Expert Review of Gastroenterology and Hepatology*. 5 (3) 411-425.

Buckley, M. 2000. Some new and important clues to the causes of colic. *British Journal of Community Nursing*. 5 (9) 462, 464-465.

Bull TJ, McMinn EJ, Sidi-Boumedine K, Skull A, Durkin D, Neild P, Rhodes G, Pickup R. and Hermon-Taylor J. 2003. Detection and verification of Mycobacterium avium subsp. paratuberculosis in fresh ileocolonic mucosal biopsy specimens from individuals with and without Crohn's disease. *Journal of Clinical Microbiology*. 41 (7) 2915-2923.

Butcher, J. 1976. The distribution of multiple sclerosis in relation to the dairy industry and milk consumption. *New Zealand Medical Journal*. 83 (566) 427-430.

Camboim Rockett F, Castro K, Rossoni de Oliveira V, da Silveira Perla A, Fagundes Chaves ML and Schweigert Perry ID. 2012. Perceived migraine triggers: do dietary factors play a role? *Nutrición hospitalaria*. 27 (2) 483-489.

Campbell TC and Campbell TM II. 2005. *The China Study*. Dallas, Texas, USA: BenBella Books.

Campbell TC and Junshi C. 1994. Diet and chronic degenerative diseases: perspectives from China. *American Journal of Clinical Nutrition*. 59 (5 Suppl) 1153S-1161S.

Campbell AK and Matthews SB. 2005. Darwin's illness revealed. *Postgraduate Medical Journal*. 81(954) 248-251.

Campbell AK, Waud JP and Matthews SB. 2009. The molecular basis of lactose intolerance. *Science Progress*. 92 (Pt 3-4) 241-287.

Campbell WW and Tang M. 2010. Protein intake, weight loss, and bone mineral density in postmenopausal women. *Journals of Gerontology. Series A Biological Sciences and Medical Sciences*. 65 (10) 1115-1122.

Cancer Research UK, 2009. *Diet and cancer: the evidence* [online]. Available from:www.cancerresearchuk.org/cancer-info/healthyliving/dietandhealthyeating/howdoweknow/diet-and-cancer-the-evidence [Accessed 27 September 2013].

Cancer Research UK, 2011. *Preventing Cancer* [online]. Available from: www.cancerresearchuk.org/cancer-help/about-cancer/causes-symptoms/preventing-cancer [Accessed 23 September 2013].

Cancer Research UK, 2012. *20 Most Common Cancers* [online]. Available from: www.cancerresearchuk.org/cancer-info/cancerstats/incidence/commoncancers/uk-cancer-incidence-statistics-for-common-cancers#Twenty [Accessed 25 September 2013].

Cancer Research UK, 2012a. *Ovarian cancer, Causes and Risks* [online]. Available from: www.cancerresearchuk.org/cancer-help/type/ovarian-cancer/about/ovarian-cancer-risks-and-causes [Accessed 7 October 2013].

Cancer Research UK, 2012b. *Prostate cancer mortality statistics* [online]. Available from: www.cancerresearchuk.org/cancer-info/cancerstats/types/prostate/mortality/uk-prostate-cancer-mortality-statistics [Accessed 9 October 2013].

Cancer Research UK, 2012c. *Prostate cancer risks and causes* [online]. Available from: www.cancerresearchuk.org/cancer-help/type/prostate-cancer/about/prostate-cancer-risks-and-causes [Accessed 9 October 2013].

Cancer Research UK, 2012d. *Prostate cancer: incidence and mortality statistics for prostate cancer worldwide*. [online]. Available from: www.cancerresearchuk.org/cancer-info/cancerstats/world/prostate-cancer-world/ [Accessed 9 October 2013].

Cancer Research UK, 2013. *All Cancers Combined* [online]. Available from: http://publications.cancerresearchuk.org/downloads/Product/CS_KF_ALLCANCERS.pdf [Accessed September 23 2013].

Cavallo MG, Fava D, Monetini L, Barone F and Pozzilli P. 1996. Cell-mediated immune response to beta casein in recent-onset insulin-dependent diabetes: implications for disease pathogenesis. *The Lancet*. 348 (9032) 926-928.

CDC, 2013. *Raw (Unpasteurized) Milk* [online]. Available from: www.cdc.gov/features/rawmilk [Accessed 14 January 2014].

Cela-Conde CJ and Ayala FJ. 2003. Genera of the human lineage. *Proceedings of the National Academy of Sciences*, 100 (13) 7684-7689.

Chan JM, Stampfer MJ, Giovannucci E, Gann PH, Ma J, Wilkinson P, Hennekens C and Pollak M. 1998. Plasma insulin-like growth factor-I and prostate cancer risk: a prospective study. *Science*. 279 (5350) 563-566.

Cho E, Spiegelman D, Hunter DJ, Chenm WY, Stampfer MJ, Colditz GA and Willett WC. 2003. Premenopausal fat intake and risk of breast cancer. *Journal of the National Cancer Institute*. 95 (14) 1079-1085.

Cho E, Smith-Warner SA, Spiegelman D, Beeson WL, van den Brandt PA, Colditz GA, Folsom AR, Fraser GE, Freudenheim JL, Giovannucci E, Goldbohm RA, Graham S, Miller AB, Pietinen P, Potter JD, Rohan TE, Terry P, Toniolo P, Virtanen MJ, Willett WC, Wolk A, Wu K, Yaun SS, Zeleniuch-Jacquotte A and Hunter DJ. 2004. Dairy foods, calcium, and colorectal cancer: a pooled analysis of 10 cohort studies. *Journal of the National Cancer Institute*. 96 (13) 1015-1022.

Cirgin Ellett ML. 2003. What is known about infant colic? *Gastroenterology Nursing*. 26 (2) 60-65.

Clarys P, Deliens T, Huybrechts I, Deriemaeker P, Vanaelst B, De Keyzer W, Hebbelinck M and Mullie P. 2014. Comparison of nutritional quality of the vegan, vegetarian, semi-vegetarian, pesco-vegetarian and omnivorous diet. *Nutrients*. 6 (3) 1318-1332.

Clein NW. 1954. Cow's milk allergy in infants. *Pediatric Clinics of North America*. 25, 949-962.

Clyne PS and Kulczycki A Jr. 1991. Human breast milk contains bovine IgG. Relationship to infant colic? *Pediatrics*. 87 (4) 439-444.

Coldham NG, Dave M, Sivapathasundaram S, McDonnell DP, Connor C. and Sauer MJ. 1997. Evaluation of a recombinant yeast cell estrogen screening assay. *Environmental Health Perspectives*. 105 (7) 734-742.

Collins MT, Lisby G, Moser C, Chicks D, Christensen S, Reichelderfer M, Hoiby N, Harms BA, Thomsen OO, Skibsted U and Binder V. 2000. Results of multiple diagnostic tests for Mycobacterium avium subsp. paratuberculosis in patients with inflammatory bowel disease and in controls. *Journal of Clinical Microbiology*. 38 (12) 4373-4381.

Copley, MS, Berstan, R, Dudd, SN, Docherty, G, Mukherjee, AJ, Straker, V, Payne, S. and Evershed, RP. 2003. Direct chemical evidence for widespread dairying in prehistoric Britain. *Proceedings of the National Academy of Sciences*, 100 (4)1524-9.

Cordain, L. 2005. Implications for the role of diet in acne. *Seminars in Cutaneous Medicine and Surgery*. 24 (2) 84-91.

da Costa PM, Loureiro L and Matos AJ. 2013. Transfer of multidrug-resistant bacteria between intermingled ecological niches: the interface between humans, animals and the environment. *International Journal of Environmental Research and Public Health*. 10 (1) 278-294.

COT, 2003. Committee on Toxicity of Chemicals in Food, Consumer Products and the Environment. *Phytoestrogens and Health*. London: The Food Standards Agency, FSA/0826/0503.

Cottet V, Touvier M, Fournier A, Touillaud MS, Lafay L, Clavel-Chapelon F and Boutron-Ruault MC. 2009. Postmenopausal breast cancer risk and dietary patterns in the E3N-EPIC prospective cohort study. *American Journal of Epidemiology*. 170 (10) 1257-1267.

Cow and Gate (careline@cowandgate.co.uk). February 11 2014. Re: *Reply from Cow and Gate*. E-mail to J. Butler (justine@viva.org.uk).

Cramer DW, Harlow BL, Willett WC, Welch WR, Bell DA, Scully RE, Ng WG and Knapp RC. 1989. Galactose consumption and metabolism in relation to the risk of ovarian cancer. *The Lancet*. 2 (8654) 66-71.

Curhan GC, Willett WC, Speizer FE, Spiegelman D and Stampfer MJ. 1997. Comparison of dietary calcium with supplemental calcium and other nutrients as factors affecting the risk for kidney stones in women. *Annals of Internal Medicine*. 126 (7) 497-504.

Curhan GC, Willett WC, Rimm EB and Stampfer MJ. 1993. A prospective study of dietary calcium and other nutrients and the risk of symptomatic kidney stones. *New England Journal of Medicine*. 328 (12) 833-838.

Daher S, Tahan S, Sole D, Naspitz CK, Da Silva, Patricio FR, Neto UF and De Morais MB. 2001. Cow's milk protein intolerance and chronic constipation in children. *Pediatric Allergy and Immunology*. 12 (6) 339-342.

Dairy Co, 2013. *UK Cow Numbers* [online] www.dairyco.org.uk/market-information/farming-data/cow-numbers/uk-cow-numbers/ [Accessed 6 September 2013].

Dairy Co, 2013a. *Average Milk Yield* [online] www.dairyco.org.uk/market-information/farming-data/milk-yield/average-milk-yield/ [Accessed 6 September 2013].

Dairy Co, 2013b. *Mastitis in Dairy Cows* [online] www.dairyco.org.uk/technical-information/animal-health-welfare/mastitis/ [Accessed 9 September 2013].

Dairy Co, 2013c. *Somatic Cell Count – Milk Quality Indicator* [online] www.dairyco.org.uk/technical-information/animal-health-welfare/mastitis/symptoms-of-mastitis/somatic-cell-count-milk-quality-indicator/ [Accessed 9 September 2013].

Dairy Co, 2013d. *Talking to the public* [online] www.dairyco.org.uk/talking-to-the-public/#.UmkdYVOJJEM [Accessed October 24 2013].

Dairy Products (Hygiene) Regulations 1995. Statutory Instrument 1995 No. 1086, London, HMSO.

D'Amico G, Gentile MG, Manna G, Fellin G, Ciceri R, Cofano F, Petrini C, Lavarda F, Perolini S and Porrini M. 1992. Effect of vegetarian soy diet on hyperlipidaemia in nephrotic syndrome. *The Lancet*. 339 (8802) 1131-1134.

Daly RM, Ebeling PR. 2010. Is excess calcium harmful to health? *Nutrients*. 2 (5) 505-522.

Danaei G, Vander Hoorn S, Lopez AD, Murray CJ, Ezzati M; Comparative Risk Assessment collaborating group (Cancers). 2005. Causes of cancer in the world: comparative risk assessment of nine behavioural and environmental risk factors. *The Lancet*. 366 (9499) 1784-1793.

Danby FW. 2005. Acne and milk, the diet myth, and beyond. *Journal of the American Academy of Dermatology*. 52 (2) 360-362.

Dargent-Molina P, Sabia S, Touvier M, Kesse E, Bréart G, Clavel-Chapelon F, Boutron-Ruault MC. 2008. Proteins, dietary acid load, and calcium and risk of postmenopausal fractures in the E3N French women prospective study. *Journal of Bone and Mineral Research*. 23 (12) 1915-1922.

Darling AL, Millward DJ, Torgerson DJ, Hewitt CE, Lanham-New SA. 2009. Dietary protein and bone health: a systematic review and meta-analysis. *American Journal of Clinical Nutrition*. 90.1674-1692.

Davenport CB. 1922. Multiple sclerosis from the standpoint of geographical distribution and race. *Archives of Neurological Psychiatry*. 8, 51-58.

Davey GK, Spencer EA, Appleby PN, Allen NE, Knox KH and Key TJ. 2003. EPIC-Oxford: lifestyle characteristics and nutrient intakes in a cohort of 33 883 meat-eaters and 31 546 non meat-eaters in the UK. *Public Health Nutrition*. 6 (3) 259-269.

Davidson RK, Jupp O, de Ferrars R, Kay CD, Culley KL, Norton R, Driscoll C, Vincent TL, Donell ST, Bao Y and Clark IM. 2013. Sulforaphane represses matrix-degrading proteases and protects cartilage from destruction in vitro and in vivo. *Arthritis and Rheumatism*. 65 (12) 130-140.

Dear KL, Compston JE and Hunter JO. 2001. Treatments for Crohn's disease that minimise steroid doses are associated with a reduced risk of osteoporosis. *Clinical Nutrition*.20 (6) 541-546.

Defra, 2012. *Agriculture in the United Kingdom 2012* [online] Available at: www.gov.uk/government/uploads/system/uploads/attachment_data/file/208436/auk-2012-25jun13.pdf [Accessed 6 September 2013].

Defra, 2013. S. Russell, Veterinary Medicines Directorate, Defra. (s.russell@vmd.defra.gsi.gov.uk) September 19 2013. *rBST query*. E-mail to J. Butler (justine@viva.org.uk).

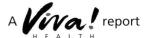

Defra, 2013a. Defra. (trade-stats@DEFRA.GSI.GOV.UK) September 30 2013. *US dairy imports query*. E-mail to J. Butler (justine@viva.org.uk).

Dehghani SM, Ahmadpour B, Haghighat M, Kashef S, Imanieh MH and Soleimani M. 2012. The Role of Cow's Milk Allergy in Pediatric Chronic Constipation: A Randomized Clinical Trial. *Iranian Journal of Pediatrics*. 22 (4) 468-474.

Department of Health, 1991. *Dietary Reference Values for Food Energy and Nutrients for the United Kingdom*. London.

Department of Health, 1994. *Weaning and the weaning diet. Report of the Working Group on the Weaning Diet of the Committee on Medical Aspects of Food Policy*. London: HMSO. Report on Health and Social Subjects No 45.

Diabetes UK, 2012. *Diabetes in the UK 2012. Key statistics on diabetes* [online]. Available from: www.diabetes.org.uk/About_us/What-we-say/Statistics/Diabetes-in-the-UK-2012/ [Accessed 17 October 2013].

Djuretic T, Wall PG and Nichols G. 1997. General outbreaks of infectious intestinal disease associated with milk and dairy products in England and Wales: 1992 to 1996. *Communicable Disease Report*. 7 (3) R41-45.

Donaldson MS. 2004. Nutrition and cancer: a review of the evidence for an anti-cancer diet. *Nutrition Journal*. 3, 19.

Doner F, Yariktas M and Demirci M. 2004. The role of allergy in recurrent otitis media with effusion. *Journal of investigational allergology and clinical immunology*. 14 (2) 154-158.

Durham WH. 1991. *Co-evolution: Genes, Culture and Human Diversity*. Stanford: Stanford University Press.

Egger J, Carter CM, Wilson J, Turner MW and Soothill JF. 1983. Is migraine food allergy? A double-blind controlled trial of oligoantigenic diet treatment. *The Lancet*. 2 (8355) 865-869.

Epstein SS. 1996. Unlabeled milk from cows treated with biosynthetic growth hormones: a case of regulatory abdication. *International Journal of Health Services*. 26 (1) 173-185.

Egro FM. 2013. Why is type 1 diabetes increasing? *Journal of Molecular Endocrinology*. 51 (1) R1-13.

El-Hodhod MA, Younis NT, Zaitoun YA and Daoud SD. 2010. Cow's milk allergy related pediatric constipation: appropriate time of milk tolerance. *Pediatric Allergy and Immunology*. 21 (2 Pt 2) e407-412.

Estep DC and Kulczycki A Jr. 2000. Colic in breast-milk-fed infants: treatment by temporary substitution of neocate infant formula. *Acta Paediatrica*. 89 (7) 795-802.

Evershed RP, Payne S, Sherratt AG, Copley MS, Coolidge J, Urem-Kotsu D, Kotsakis K, Ozdoğan M, Ozdoğan AE, Nieuwenhuyse O, Akkermans PM, Bailey D, Andeescu RR, Campbell S, Farid S, Hodder I, Yalman N, Ozbaşaran M, Biçakci E, Garfinkel Y, Levy T and Burton MM. 2008. Earliest date for milk use in the Near East and southeastern Europe linked to cattle herding. *Nature*. 455 (7212) 528-531.

Faber MT, Jensen A, Søgaard M, Høgdall E, Høgdall C, Blaakaer J and Kjaer SK. 2012. Use of dairy products, lactose, and calcium and risk of ovarian cancer - results from a Danish case-control study. *Acta Oncologica*. 51 (4) 454-464.

Fairfield KM, Hunter DJ, Colditz GA, Fuchs CS, Cramer DW, Speizer FE, Willett WC and Hankinson SE. 2004. A prospective study of dietary lactose and ovarian cancer. *International Journal of Cancer*. 110 (2) 271-277.

FAO, 1997. Latham, M.C. *Human nutrition in the developing world*. Rome: FAO Food and Nutrition Series No. 29. Cornell University Ithaca, New York, USA.

FAO, 2009. *The State of Food and Agriculture* [online]. Available from: www.fao.org/docrep/012/i0680e/i0680e.pdf [Accessed 9 September 2012].

FAOSTAT, 2013. *Food Supply* [online] Available at: http://faostat.fao.org/site/610/DesktopDefault.aspx?PageID=610#ancor [Accessed 6 September 2013].

Farlow DW, Xu X and Veenstra TD. 2009. Quantitative measurement of endogenous estrogen metabolites, risk-factors for development of breast cancer, in commercial milk products by LC-MS/MS. *Journal of Chromatography. B Analytical Technologies in the Biomedical and Life Sciences*. 877 (13) 1327-1334.

Farooq S and Coleman MP. 2005. Breast cancer survival in South Asian women in England and Wales. *Journal of Epidemiology and Community Health*. 59 (5) 402-406.

Feskanich D, Willett WC, Stampfer MJ and Colditz GA. 1997. Milk, dietary calcium, and bone fractures in women: a 12-year prospective study. *The American Journal of Public Health*. 87 (6) 992-997.

Fey PD, Safranek TJ, Rupp ME, Dunne EF, Ribot E, Iwen PC, Bradford PA, Angulo FJ. and Hinrichs SH. 2000. Ceftriaxone-resistant salmonella infection acquired by a child from cattle. *New England Journal of Medicine* 342 (17) 1242-1249.

FDA, 1999. Food labeling health claims: soy protein and coronary heart disease. Food and Drug Administration, HHS. Final rule. *Federal Register*. 64, 57700-57733.

Fenton TR, Lyon AW, Eliasziw M, Tough SC and Hanley DA. 2009. Meta-analysis of the effect of the acid-ash hypothesis of osteoporosis on calcium balance. *Journal of Bone and Mineral Research*. 24 (11) 1835-1840.

Fenton TR, Tough SC, Lyon AW, Eliasziw M and Hanley DA. 20011. Causal assessment of dietary acid load and bone disease: a systematic review & meta-analysis applying Hill's epidemiologic criteria for causality. *Nutrition Journal*. 10:41.

Fraser GE. 1999. Associations between diet and cancer, ischemic heart disease, and all-cause mortality in non-Hispanic white California Seventh-day Adventists. *American Journal of Clinical Nutrition*. 70 (3 Supplement) 532S-538S.

Fraser GE. 2009. Vegetarian diets: what do we know of their effects on common chronic diseases? *American Journal of Clinical Nutrition*. 89 (Suppl) 1607S-1612S.

Frassetto LA, Todd KM, Morris RC Jr and Sebastian A. 2000. Worldwide incidence of hip fracture in elderly women: relation to consumption of animal and vegetable foods. *The Journals of Gerontology. Series A, Biological Sciences and Medical Sciences*. 55 (10) M585-592.

Frassetto LA, Morris RC Jr, Sellmeyer DE and Sebastian A. 2008. Adverse effects of sodium chloride on bone in the aging human population resulting from habitual consumption of typical American diets. *Journal of Nutrition*. 138 (2) 419S-422S.

Frassetto LA and Sebastian A. 2013. Commentary to accompany the paper entitled 'nutritional disturbance in acid-base balance and osteoporosis: a hypothesis that disregards the essential homeostatic role of the kidney', by Jean-Philippe Bonjour. *British Journal of Nutrition*. 110 (11) 1935-1937.

Frye JG and Jackson CR. 2013. Genetic mechanisms of antimicrobial resistance identified in Salmonella enterica, Escherichia coli, and Enteroccocus spp. isolated from U.S. food animals. *Frontiers in Microbiology*. 4:135.

FSA/SE, 2001. *Task force on E. coli O157* [online] Available at: www.food.gov.uk/multimedia/pdfs/ecolitaskfinreport.pdf [Accessed 15 October 2013].

FSA, 2002. McCance and Widdowson's *The Composition of Foods, 6th summary edition*. Cambridge, England, Royal Society of Chemistry.

FSA, 2002a. *A review of the evidence for a link between exposure to Mycobacterium paratuberculosis (MAP) and Crohn's disease (CD) in humans*. A report for the Food Standards Agency January 2002. [online] Available from: www.food.gov.uk/multimedia/pdfs/mapcrohnreport.pdf [Accessed 16 October 2013].

FSA, 2003. *Strategy for the control of Mycobacterium avium subspecies paratuberculosis (MAP) in cow's milk*. [online] Available from: www.food.gov.uk/multimedia/pdfs/map_strategy.pdf [Accessed 16 October 2013].

FSA, 2006. *Second progress report on strategy for the control of mycobacterium avium subspecies paratuberculosis (MAP) in cows' milk* [online]. http://tna.europarchive.org/20130814101929/ http://www.food.gov.uk/multimedia/pdfs/int060311rev1.pdf [Accessed 15 October 2013].

FSA, 2009. *Raw drinking milk and raw cream control requirements in the different countries of the UK* [online]. www.food.gov.uk/business-industry/guidancenotes/dairy-guidance/rawmilkcream [Accessed 14 January 2014].

FSA, 2013. *Measuring foodborne illness levels* [online]. www.food.gov.uk/policy-advice/microbiology/fds/ 58736#.UmRT4VOJJEM [Accessed 15 October 2013].

FSA, 2013a. *Annual Report of the Chief Scientist 2012/13* [online]. www.food.gov.uk/multimedia/pdfs/publication/cstar_2013.pdf [Accessed 20 October 2013].

Fuchs CS, Giovannucci EL, Colditz GA, Hunter DJ, Stampfer MJ, Rosner B, Speizer FE and Willett WC. 1999. Dietary fiber and the risk of colorectal cancer and adenoma in women. *New England Journal of Medicine*. 340 (3) 169-176.

Ganmaa D and Sato A. 2005. The possible role of female sex hormones in milk from pregnant cows in the development of breast, ovarian and corpus uteri cancers. *Medical Hypotheses*. 65 (6) 1028-1037.

Garland CF, Garland FC and Gorham ED. 1999. Calcium and vitamin D. Their potential roles in colon and breast cancer prevention. *Annals of the New York Academy of Sciences*. 889, 107-119.

Genkinger JM, Platz EA, Hoffman SC, Comstock GW and Helzlsouer KJ. 2004. Fruit, vegetable, and antioxidant intake and all-cause, cancer, and cardiovascular disease mortality in a community-dwelling population in Washington County, Maryland. *American Journal of Epidemiology*. 160 (12) 1223-1233.

Gerber M. 1998. Fibre and breast cancer. *European Journal of Cancer Prevention*. 7 Supplement 2, S63-67.

German JB, Dillard CJ and Ward RE. 2002. Bioactive components in milk. *Current Opinion in Clinical Nutrition and Metabolic Care*. 5 (6) 653-658.

Gerstein HC. 1994. Cow's milk exposure and type I diabetes mellitus. A critical overview of the clinical literature. *Diabetes Care*. 17 (1) 13-9.

Gillespie KM, Bain SC, Barnett AH, Bingley PJ, Christie MR, Gill GV and Gale EA. 2004. The rising incidence of childhood type 1 diabetes and reduced contribution of high-risk HLA haplotypes. *Lancet*. 364 (9446) 1699-700.

Giovannucci E. 1998. Dietary influences of 1,25(OH)2 vitamin D in relation to prostate cancer: a hypothesis. *Cancer Causes Control*. 9 (6) 567-582.

Giovanucci E, Rimm EB, Wolk A, Ascherio A, Stampfer MJ, Colditz GA and Willett WC. 1998a. Calcium and fructose in relation to risk of prostate cancer. *Cancer Research*. 58 (3) 442-447.

Giovannucci E, Pollak MN, Platz EA, Willett WC, Stampfer MJ, Majeed N, Colditz GA, Speizer FE and Hankinson SE. 2000. A prospective study of plasma insulin-like growth factor-1 and binding protein-3 and risk of colorectal neoplasia in women. *Cancer Epidemiology, Biomarkers and Prevention: a publication of the American Association for Cancer Research, cosponsored by the American Society of Preventive Oncology*. 9 (4) 345-349.

Glantz, S and Gonzalez, M. 2012. Effective tobacco control is key to rapid progress in reduction of non-communicable diseases. *Lancet*. 379 (9822) 1269-1271.

Greer FR and Krebs NF; American Academy of Pediatrics Committee on Nutrition. Optimizing bone health and calcium intakes of infants, children, and adolescents. 2006. *Pediatrics*. 117 (2) 578-585.

Grosvenor CE, Picciano MF and Baumrucker CR. 1992. Hormones and growth factors in milk. *Endocrine Reviews*. 14 (6) 710-728.

Gunnell D, Oliver SE, Peters TJ, Donovan JL, Persad R, Maynard M, Gillatt D, Pearce A, Hamdy FC, Neal DE and Holly JM. 2003. Are diet-prostate cancer associations mediated by the IGF axis? A cross-sectional analysis of diet, IGF-I and IGFBP-3 in healthy middle-aged men. *British Journal of Cancer*. 88 (11) 1682-6.

Gunther CW, Legowski PA, Lyle RM, McCabe GP, Eagan MS, Peacock M and Teegarden D. 2005. Dairy products do not lead to alterations in body weight or fat mass in young women in a 1-y intervention. *American Journal of Clinical Nutrition*. 81 (4) 751-756.

Gustafson D, Rothenberg E, Blennow K, Steen B and Skoog I. 2003. An 18-year follow-up of overweight and risk of Alzheimer's disease. *Archives of Internal Medicine*. 163 (13) 1524-1528.

Hafstrom I, Ringertz B, Spangberg A, von Zweigbergk L, Brannemark S, Nylander I, Ronnelid J, Laasonen L and Klareskog L. 2001. A vegan diet free of gluten improves the signs and symptoms of rheumatoid arthritis: the effects on arthritis correlate with a reduction in antibodies to food antigens. *Rheumatology* (Oxford). 40 (10) 1175-1179.

Hall B, Chesters J and Robinson A. 2012. Infantile colic: a systematic review of medical and conventional therapies. *Paediatric Child Health*. 48 (2) 128-137.

Hamlyn B, Brooker S, Oleinikova K and Wands S. 2002. *Infant Feeding 2000*. The Stationery Office. London, UK.

Hammerum AM and Heuer OE. 2009. Human health hazards from antimicrobial-resistant *Escherichia coli* of animal origin. *Clinical Infectious Diseases*. 48(7):916-21

Hankinson SE, Willett WC, Manson JE, Colditz GA, Hunter DJ, Spiegelman D, Barbieri RL and Speizer FE. 1998. Plasma sex steroid hormone levels and risk of breast cancer in postmenopausal women. *Journal of the National Cancer Institute*. 90 (17) 1292-1299.

Hankinson SE, Willett WC, Colditz GA, Hunter DJ, Michaud DS, Deroo B, Rosner B, Speizer FE and Pollak M. 1998a. Circulating concentrations of insulin-like growth factor-I and risk of breast cancer. *The Lancet*. 351, 1393-1396.

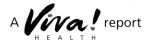

Harder T, Bergmann R, Kallischnigg G and Plagemann A. 2005. Duration of breastfeeding and risk of overweight: a meta-analysis. *American Journal of Epidemiology*. 162, 397-403.

Harrington LK and Mayberry JF. 2008. A re-appraisal of lactose intolerance. *International Journal of Clinical Practice*. 62 (10) 1541-1546.

Harvey-Berino J, Gold BC, Lauber R and Starinski A. 2005. The impact of calcium and dairy product consumption on weight loss. *Obesity Research*. 13 (10) 1720-1726.

He FJ, Nowson CA, Lucas M and MacGregor GA. 2007. Increased consumption of fruit and vegetables is related to a reduced risk of coronary heart disease: meta-analysis of cohort studies. *Journal of Human Hypertension*. 21 (9) 717-728.

Heaney RP, McCarron DA, Dawson-Hughes B, Oparil S, Berga SL, Stern JS, Barr SI and Rosen CJ. 1999. Dietary changes favourably affect bone remodelling in older adults. *Journal of the American Dietetic Association*. 99 (10) 1228-1233.

Heaney RP and Weaver CM. 1990. Calcium absorption from kale. *American Journal of Clinical Nutrition*. 51 (4) 656-657.

Heaney RP. 2002. Protein and calcium: antagonists or synergists? *American Journal of Clinical Nutrition*. 75 (4) 609-610.

Henderson L, Gregory J, Irving K, and Swan G. 2003. *National Diet and Nutrition Survey: adults aged 19 to 64 years: Energy, protein, carbohydrate, fat and alcohol intake*. London: TSO. Volume 2.

Henderson L, Irving K, Gregory J, Bates CJ, Prentice A, Perks J, Swan G and Farron, M. 2003a. *National Diet and Nutrition Survey: adults aged 19 to 64 years: Vitamin and mineral intake and urinary analytes*. London: TSO. Volume 3.

Hermann R, Knip M, Veijola R, Simell O, Laine AP, Akerblom HK, Groop PH, Forsblom C, Pettersson-Fernholm K, Ilonen J; FinnDiane Study Group. 2003. Temporal changes in the frequencies of HLA genotypes in patients with Type 1 diabetes--indication of an increased environmental pressure? *Diabetologia*. 46 (3) 420-425.

Hermon-Taylor J. 2009. Mycobacterium avium subspecies paratuberculosis, Crohn's disease and the Doomsday scenario. *Gut Pathology*. 1 (1) 15.

Hex N, Bartlett C, Wright D, Taylor M and Varley D. 2012. Estimating the current and future costs of Type 1 and Type 2 diabetes in the UK, including direct health costs and indirect societal and productivity costs. *Diabetic Medicine*. 29 (7) 855-862.

Heyman MB. 2006. Lactose intolerance in infants, children, and adolescents. *Pediatrics*. 118 (3) 1279-1286.

Hill, LW and Stuart HC. 1929. A soya bean food preparation for feeding infants with milk idiosyncrasy. *Journal of the American Medical Association*. 93, 985-987.

Hoffman JR and Falvo MJ. 2004. Protein – Which is Best? *Journal of Sports Science and Medicine*. (3) 118-130.

Holly, 2013. Professor Jeff Holly (jeff.holly@bristol.ac.uk) September 2 2013. *IGF-1 and dairy consumption*. E-mail to J. Butler (justine@viva.org.uk).

Holly JM, Zeng L and Perks CM. 2013. Epithelial cancers in the post-genomic era: should we reconsider our lifestyle? *Cancer Metastasis Reviews*. Aug 2. [Epub ahead of print]

Holmes MD, Pollak MN, Willett WC and Hankinson SE. 2002. Dietary correlates of plasma insulin-like growth factor 1 and insulin-like growth factor binding protein 3 concentrations. *Cancer Epidemiology Biomarkers and Prevention*. 11 (9) 852-861.

Honegger A and Humbel RE. 1986. Insulin-like growth factors I and II in fetal and adult bovine serum. Purification, primary structures, and immunological cross-reactivities. *Journal of Biological Chemistry*. 26, 569-575.

Hoppe C, Udam TR, Lauritzen L, Molgaard C, Juul A and Michaelsen KF. 2004. Animal protein intake, serum insulin-like growth factor I, and growth in healthy 2.5-y-old Danish children. *American Journal of Clinical Nutrition*. 80 (2) 447-452.

Hoppu U, Kalliomaki M and Isolauri E. 2000. Maternal diet rich in saturated fat during breastfeeding is associated with atopic sensitization of the infant. *European Journal of Clinical Nutrition*. 54 (9) 702-705.

Hoppu U, Rinne M, Lampi AM and Isolauri E. 2005. Breast milk fatty acid composition is associated with development of atopic dermatitis in the infant. *Journal of Pediatric Gastroenterology and Nutrition*. 41 (3) 335-338.

Howe GR, Hirohata T, Hislop TG, Iscovich JM, Yuan JM, Katsouyanni K, Lubin F, Marubini E, Modan B, Rohan T, Toniolo P and Shunxhang Y. 1990. Dietary factors and risk of breast cancer: combined analysis of 12 case-control studies. *Journal of the National Cancer Institute*. 82 (7) 561-569.

Hu FB, Manson JE and Willett WC 2001. Types of dietary fat and risk of coronary heart disease: a critical review. *Journal of the American College of Nutrition*. 20 (1) 5-19.

Huncharek M, Muscat J and Kupelnick B. 2009. Colorectal cancer risk and dietary intake of calcium, vitamin D, and dairy products: a meta-analysis of 26,335 cases from 60 observational studies. *Nutrition and Cancer*. 61 (1) 47-69.

Hurst DS. 1998. *The relation of allergy to otitis media with effusion: clinical and histochemical studies*. Uppsala University, Sweden: Acta Universitatis Upsaliensis.

Iacobucci G. 2013. UK has fifth highest rate of type 1 diabetes in children, new figures show. *British Medical Journal*. 3; 346: f22.

IARC, 1997. *Cancer incidence in five continents*. Volume VII. International Agency for Research on Cancer (IARC) Scientific Publications. 143: i-xxxiv, 1-1240.

Iacono G, Cavataio F, Montalto G, Florena A, Tumminello M, Soresi M, Notarbartolo A and Carroccio A. 1998. Intolerance of cow's milk and chronic constipation in children. *New England Journal of Medicine*. 339 (16) 1100-1104.

ISAAC. 1998. The International Study of Asthma and Allergies in Childhood (ISAAC) Steering Committee. Worldwide variation in prevalence of symptoms of asthma, allergic rhinoconjunctivitis, and atopic eczema. *The Lancet*. 351, 1225-1232.

Ishida BK and Chapman MH. 2004. A comparison of carotenoid content and total antioxidant activity in catsup from several commercial sources in the United States. *Journal of Agricultural and Food Chemistry*. 52 (26) 8017-8020.

Jacobs DR Jr, Marquart L, Slavin J and Kushi LH. 1998. Whole-grain intake and cancer: an expanded review and meta-analysis. *Nutrition and Cancer*. 30 (2) 85-96.

Jakobsson I and Lindberg T. 1978. Cow's milk as a cause of infantile colic in breast-fed infants. *The Lancet*. 2 (8092 Pt 1) 734.

Jakobsson I and Lindberg T. 1983. Cow's milk proteins cause infantile colic in breast-fed infants: a double-blind crossover study. *Pediatrics*. 71 (2) 268-271.

Jakobsson I, Lothe L, Ley D and Borschel MW. 2000. Effectiveness of casein hydrolysate feedings in infants with colic. *Acta Paediatrica*. 89 (1) 18-21.

James JM, Bernhisel-Broadbent J and Sampson HA. 1994. Respiratory reactions provoked by double-blind food challenges in children. *American Journal of Respiratory and Critical Care Medicine*. 149, 59-64.

James JM. 2004. Common respiratory manifestations of food allergy: a critical focus on otitis media. *Current Allergy and Asthma Reports*. 4 (4) 294-301.

James DC and Lessen R; American Dietetic Association. 2009. Position of the American Dietetic Association: promoting and supporting breastfeeding. *Journal of the American Dietetic Association*. 109 (11) 1926-1942.

Janisiewicz WJ, Conway WS, Brown MW, Sapers GM, Fratamico P and Buchanan RL. 1999. Fate of Escherichia coli O157:H7 on fresh-cut apple tissue and its potential for transmission by fruit flies. *Applied Environmental Microbiology*. 65 (1) 1-5.

Jenkins DJ, Mirrahimi A, Srichaikul K, Berryman CE, Wang L, Carleton A, Abdulnour S, Sievenpiper JL, Kendall CW and Kris-Etherton PM. 2010. Soy protein reduces serum cholesterol by both intrinsic and food displacement mechanisms. *Journal of Nutrition*. 140 (12) 2302S-2311S.

Jha V, Garcia-Garcia G, Iseki K, Li Z, Naicker S, Plattner B, Saran R, Wang AY and Yang CW. 2013. Chronic kidney disease: global dimension and perspectives. *Lancet*. 382 (9888) 260-272.

JHCI, 2002. *Joint Health Claims Initiative*. [online] Available from: http://webarchive.nationalarchives.gov.uk/nobanner/20130404135254/http://www.jhci.org.uk/approv/schol2.htm [Accessed 11 February 2014).

Juntti H, Tikkanen S, Kokkonen J, Alho OP and Niinimaki A. 1999. Cow's milk allergy is associated with recurrent otitis media during childhood. *Acta Oto-laryngologica*. 119 (8) 867-873.

Kaaks R, Toniolo P, Akhmedkhanov A, Lukanova A, Biessy C, Dechaud H, Rinaldi S, Zeleniuch-Jacquotte A, Shore RE and Riboli E. 2000. Serum C-peptide, insulin-like growth factor (IGF)-I, IGF-binding proteins, and colorectal cancer risk in women. *Journal of the National Cancer Institute*. 92 (19) 1592-1600.

Kanis JA, Odén A, McCloskey EV, Johansson H, Wahl DA and Cooper C; IOF Working Group on Epidemiology and Quality of Life. 2012. A systematic review of hip fracture incidence and probability of fracture worldwide. *Osteoporosis International*. 23 (9) 2239-2256.

Kannel WB, Dawber TR, Kagan A, Revotskiw N and Stokes J 3rd. 1961. Factors of risk in the development of coronary heart disease--six year follow-up experience. The Framingham Study. *Annals of Internal Medicine*. 55, 33-50.

Karjalainen J, Martin JM, Knip M, Ilonen J, Robinson BH, Savilahti E, Akerblom HK and Dosch HM. 1992. A bovine albumin peptide as a possible trigger of insulin-dependent diabetes mellitus. *New England Journal of Medicine*. 327 (5) 302-307.

Kerstetter JE, O'Brien KO and Insogna KL. 2003. Dietary protein, calcium metabolism, and skeletal homeostasis revisited. *American Journal of Clinical Nutrition*. 78 (3 Suppl) 584S-592S.

Kerstetter JE, O'Brien KO, Caseria DM, Wall DE, Insogna KL. 2005. The impact of dietary protein on calcium absorption and kinetic measures of bone turnover in women. *The Journal of Clinical Endocrinology and Metabolism*. 90 (1) 26-31.

Key TJ, Davey GK and Appleby PN. 1999. Health benefits of a vegetarian diet. *Proceedings of the Nutrition Society*. 58 (2) 271-275.

Key TJ, Fraser GE, Thorogood M, Appleby PN, Beral V, Reeves G, Burr ML, Chang-Claude J, Frentzel-Beyme R, Kuzma JW, Mann J and McPherson K. 1999. Mortality in vegetarians and nonvegetarians: detailed findings from a collaborative analysis of 5 prospective studies. *American Journal of Clinical Nutrition*. 70 (Suppl) 516S-524S.

Key TJ, Appleby PN, Spencer EA, Roddam AW, Neale RE and Allen NE. 2007. Calcium, diet and fracture risk: a prospective study of 1,898 incident fractures among 34,696 British women and men. *Public Health Nutrition*. 10 (11) 1314-1320.

Key TJ, Appleby PN, Spencer EA, Travis RC, Allen NE, Thorogood M and Mann JI. 2009. Cancer incidence in British vegetarians. *British Journal of Cancer*. 101:192–197.

Key TJ, Appleby PH, Spencer EA, Travis RC, Roddam AW and Allen NE. 2009a. Cancer incidence in vegetarians: results from the European Prospective Investigation in Cancer and Nutrition (EPIC-Oxford). *American Journal of Clinical Nutrition*. 89 (Suppl) :1620S-1626S.

Key TJ, Appleby PN, Reeves GK, Roddam AW, Helzlsouer KJ, Alberg AJ, Rollison DE, Dorgan JF, Brinton LA, Overvad K, Kaaks R, Trichopoulou A, Clavel-Chapelon F, Panico S, Duell EJ, Peeters PH, Rinaldi S, Fentiman IS, Dowsett M, Manjer J, Lenner P, Hallmans G, Baglietto L, English DR, Giles GG, Hopper JL, Severi G, Morris HA, Hankinson SE, Tworoger SS, Koenig K, Zeleniuch-Jacquotte A, Arslan AA, Toniolo P, Shore RE, Krogh V, Micheli A, Berrino F, Barrett-Connor E, Laughlin GA, Kabuto M, Akiba S, Stevens RG, Neriishi K, Land CE, Cauley JA, Lui LY, Cummings SR, Gunter MJ, Rohan TE and Strickler HD. Endogenous Hormones and Breast Cancer Collaborative Group. 2011. Circulating sex hormones and breast cancer risk factors in postmenopausal women: reanalysis of 13 studies. *British Journal of Cancer*. 105 (5) 709-722.

Key TJ, Appleby PN, Cairns BJ, Luben R, Dahm CC, Akbaraly T, Brunner EJ, Burley V, Cade JE, Greenwood DC, Stephen AM, Mishra G, Kuh D, Keogh RH, White IR, Bhaniani A, Borgulya G, Mulligan AA and Khaw KT. 2011a. Dietary fat and breast cancer: comparison of results from food diaries and food-frequency questionnaires in the UK Dietary Cohort Consortium. *American Journal of Clinical Nutrition*. 94 (4) 1043-1052.

Key TJ, Appleby PN, Crowe FL, Bradbury KE, Schmidt JA andTravis RC. 2014. Cancer in British vegetarians: updated analyses of 4998 incident cancers in a cohort of 32,491 meat eaters, 8612 fish eaters, 18,298 vegetarians, and 2246 vegans. *American Journal of Clinical Nutrition*. June 4; 100 (Supplement 1) :378S-385S.

Kimpimaki T, Erkkola M, Korhonen S, Kupila A, Virtanen SM., Ilonen J, Simell O and Knip M. 2001. Short-term exclusive breastfeeding predisposes young children with increased genetic risk of Type I diabetes to progressive beta-cell autoimmunity. *Diabetologia*. 44 (1) 63-69.

Klein KO. 1998. Isoflavones, soy-based infant formulas, and relevance to endocrine function. *Nutrition Review*. 56 (7) 193-204.

Krajcovicova-Kudlackova M, Babinska K and Valachovicova M. 2005. Health benefits and risks of plant proteins. *Bratislavske Lekarske Listy*. 106 (6-7) 231-234.

Kucuk O, Sarkar FH, Sakr W, Djuric Z, Pollak MN, Khachik F, Li YW, Banerjee M, Grignon D, Bertram JS, Crissman JD, Pontes EJ and Wood DP Jr. 2001. Phase II randomized clinical trial of lycopene supplementation before radical prostatectomy. *Cancer Epidemiology Biomarkers and Prevention*. 10 (8) 861-868.

Lanou AJ. 2005. Data do not support recommending dairy products for weight loss. *Obesity Research*. 13 (1) 191.

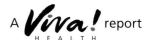

Lanou AJ, Berkow SE and Barnard ND. 2005. Calcium, Dairy Products, and Bone Health in Children and Young Adults: A Re-evaluation of the Evidence. *Pediatrics*. 115 (3) 736-743.

Lanou AJ. 2006 Oct Bone health in children. *The British Medical Journal*. 14; 333 (7572) 763-764.

Lanou AJ and Svenson B. 2010. Reduced cancer risk in vegetarians: an analysis of recent reports. *Cancer Management and Research*. 3:1-8.

Lappe JM, Rafferty KA, Davies KM and Lypaczewski G. 2004 . Girls on a high-calcium diet gain weight at the same rate as girls on a normal diet: a pilot study. *Journal of the American Dietetic Association*. 104 (9) 1361-1367.

van de Laar MA and van der Korst JK. 1992. Food intolerance in rheumatoid arthritis. I. A double blind, controlled trial of the clinical effects of elimination of milk allergens and azo dyes. *Annals of the Rheumatic Diseases*. 51 (3) 298-302.

Larsson SC, Bergkvist L and Wolk A. 2004. Milk and lactose intakes and ovarian cancer risk in the Swedish Mammography Cohort. *American Journal of Clinical Nutrition*. 80 (5) 1353-1357.

Larsson SC, Orsini N and Wolk A. 2006. 2006. Milk, milk products and lactose intake and ovarian cancer risk: a meta-analysis of epidemiological studies. *International Journal of Cancer*. 118 (2) 431-441.

Lasekan JB, Ostrom KM, Jacobs JR, Blatter MM, Ndife LI, Gooch WM 3rd and Cho S. 1999. Growth of newborn, term infants fed soy formulas for one year. *Clinical Pediatrics*. 38 (10) 563-571.

Lees B, Molleson T, Arnett TR and Stevenson JC. 1993. Differences in proximal femur bone density over two centuries. *The Lancet*. 13, 341 (8846) 673-675.

Lehtonen L, Korvenranta H and Eerola E. 1994. Intestinal microflora in colicky and noncolicky infants: bacterial cultures and gas-liquid chromatography. *Journal of Pediatric Gastroenterology and Nutrition*. 19 (3) 310-314.

Leitzmann C. 2005. Vegetarian diets: what are the advantages? *Forum of Nutrition*. (57) 147-56.

LeRoith D, Werner H, Neuenschwander S, Kalebic T and Helman LJ. 1995. The role of the insulin-like growth factor-I receptor in cancer. *Annals of the New York Academy of Sciences*. 766, 402-408.

Lewin MH, Bailey N, Bandaletova T, Bowman R, Cross AJ, Pollock J, Shuker DE and Bingham SA. 2006. Red meat enhances the colonic formation of the DNA adduct O6-carboxymethyl guanine: implications for colorectal cancer risk. *Cancer Research*. 66 (3) 1859-1865.

Lindberg T. 1999. Infantile colic and small intestinal function: a nutritional problem? *Acta Paediatrica Suppl*. 88 (430) 58-60.

Linnan MJ, Mascola L, Lou XD, Goulet V, May S, Salminen C, Hird DW, Yonekura ML, Hayes P and Weaver R. 1988. Epidemic listeriosis associated with Mexican-style cheese. *New England Journal of Medicine*. 29, 319 (13) 823-828.

Lipsitch M, Singer RS and Levin BR 2002. Antibiotics in agriculture: When is it time to close the barn door? *Proceedings of the National Academy of Sciences*. 99, 5752-5754.

Little CL, Pires SM, Gillespie IA, Grant K and Nichols GL. 2010. Attribution of human Listeria monocytogenes infections in England and Wales to ready-to-eat food sources placed on the market: adaptation of the Hald Salmonella source attribution model. *Foodborne Pathogenic Diseases*. 7 (7) 749-756.

Lloyd T, Petit MA, Lin HM and Beck TJ. 2004. Lifestyle factors and the development of bone mass and bone strength in young women. *The Journal of Pediatrics*. 144 (6) 776-782.

Lock AL and Garnsworthy PC. 2002. Independent effects of dietary linoleic and linolenic fatty acids on the conjugated linoleic acid content of cows' milk. *Animal Science*. 74, 63-176.

Loef M and Walach H. 2013. Midlife obesity and dementia: meta-analysis and adjusted forecast of dementia prevalence in the United States and China. *Obesity (Silver Spring)*. 21 (1) E51-55.

Lomer MC, Parkes GC and Sanderson JD. 2008. Review article: lactose intolerance in clinical practice--myths and realities. *Alimentary Pharmacology and Therapeutics*. 27 (2) 193-103.

Lothe L and Lindberg T. 1989. Cow's milk whey protein elicits symptoms of infantile colic in colicky formula-fed infants: a double-blind crossover study. *Pediatrics*. 83 (2) 262-266.

Lovati MR, Manzoni C, Canavesi A, Sirtori M, Vaccarino V, Marchi M, Gaddi G and Sirtori, CR. 1987. Soybean protein diet increases low density lipoprotein receptor activity in mononuclear cells from hypercholesterolemic patients. *The Journal of Clinical Investigation*. 80 (5) 1498-1502.

Lovati MR, Manzoni C, Gianazza E, Arnoldi A, Kurowska E, Carroll KK and Sirtori CR. 2000. Soy protein peptides regulate cholesterol homeostasis in Hep G2 cells. *Journal of Nutrition*. 130 (10) 2543-2549.

Lucassen PL, Assendelft WJ, Gubbels JW, van Eijk JT, van Geldrop WJ and Neven AK. 1998. Effectiveness of treatments for infantile colic: systematic review. *British Medical Journal*. 316 (7144) 1563-1569.

Lucassen PL, Assendelft WJ, Gubbels JW, van Eijk JT and Douwes AC. 2000. Infantile colic: crying time reduction with a whey hydrolysate: A double-blind, randomized, placebo-controlled trial. *Pediatrics*. 106 (6) 1349-1354.

Lust KD, Brown E and Thomas W. 1996. Maternal intake of cruciferous vegetables and other foods and colic symptoms in exclusively breast-fed infants. *Journal of the American Dietetic Association*. 96 (1) 46-48.

Ma J, Pollak MN, Giovannucci E, Chan JM, Tao Y, Hennekens CH. and Stampfer M.J. 1999. Prospective study of colorectal cancer risk in men and plasma levels of insulin-like growth factor (IGF)-I and IGF-binding protein-3. *Journal of the National Cancer Institute*. 91 (7) 620-625.

Macmillan Cancer Support, 2011. *Breast cancer risk factors and causes* [online]. Available from: www.macmillan.org.uk/Cancerinformation/Cancertypes/Breast/Aboutbreastcancer/Causes.aspx#DynamicJumpMenuManager_5_Anchor_5 [Accessed 25 September 2013].

Macmillan Cancer Support, 2013. *By 2020 almost half of Britons will get cancer in their lifetime – but 38% will not die from the disease* [online]. Available from: www.macmillan.org.uk/Aboutus/News/Latest_News/By2020almosthalfofBritonswillgetcancerintheirlifetime%E2%80%93but38willnotdiefromthedisease.aspx [Accessed 23 September 2013].

Macmillan Cancer Support, 2013a. *Cancer genetics - prostate cancer* [online]. Available from: www.macmillan.org.uk/Cancerinformation/Causesriskfactors/Genetics/Cancergenetics/Specificconditions/Prostatecancer.aspx [Accessed 10 October 2013].

Malosse D, Perron H, Sasco A and Seigneurin JM. 1992. Correlation between milk and dairy product consumption and multiple sclerosis prevalence: a worldwide study. *Neuroepidemiology*. 11 (4-6) 304-312.

Marsh AG, Sanchez TV, Michelsen O, Chaffee FL and Fagal SM. 1988. Vegetarian lifestyle and bone mineral density. *American Journal of Clinical Nutrition*. 48 (3 Supplement) 837-841.

Martin JM, Trink B, Daneman D, Dosch HM and Robinson B. 1991. Milk proteins in the etiology of insulin-dependent diabetes mellitus (IDDM). *Annals of Medicine*. 23 (4) 447-452.

Martinez GA, Ryan AS and Malec DJ. 1985. Nutrient intakes of American infants and children fed cow's milk or infant formula. *American Journal of Diseases in Children*. 139 (10) 1010-1018.

Massey LK. 2003. Dietary animal and plant protein and human bone health: a whole foods approach. *Journal of Nutrition*. 133 (3) 862S-865S.

Matthews SB, Waud JP, Roberts AG and Campbell AK. 2005. Systemic lactose intolerance: a new perspective on an old problem. *Postgraduate Medical Journal*. 81 (953) 167-173.

Mattisson I, Wirfält E, Johansson U, Gullberg B, Olsson H, Berglund G. 2004. Intakes of plant foods, fibre and fat and risk of breast cancer--a prospective study in the Malmö Diet and Cancer cohort. *British Journal of Cancer*. 90 (1) 122-127.

Mazess RB and Mather WE. 1974. Bone mineral content of North Alaskan Eskimos. *American Journal of Clinical Nutrition*. 27 (9) 916-25.

Mazess RB and Mather WE. 1975. Bone mineral content in Canadian Eskimos. *Human Biology*. 47 (1) 44-63.

McCormack VA, Mangtani P, Bhakta D, McMichael AJ and dos Santos Silva I. 2004. Heterogeneity of breast cancer risk within the South Asian female population in England: a population-based case-control study of first-generation migrants. *British Journal of Cancer*. 90 (1) 160-166.

McGuire MA and McGuire MK. 2000. Conjugated linoleic acid (CLA): A ruminant fatty acid with beneficial effects on human health. (Invited Review). *Proceedings of the American Society of Animal Science*. [online] Available from: www.asas.org/jas/symposia/proceedings/0938.pdf [Accessed 6 March 2006].

McCrorie TA, Keaveney EM, Wallace JM, Binns N and Livingstone MB. 2011 Human health effects of conjugated linoleic acid from milk and supplements. *Nutrition Research Reviews*. 24 (2) 206-227.

McDougall J, Bruce B, Spiller G, Westerdahl J and McDougall M. 2002. Effects of a very low-fat, vegan diet in subjects with rheumatoid arthritis. *Journal of Alternative Complementary Medicine*. 8 (1) 71-75.

Meinbach DS and Lokeshwar BL. 2006. Insulin-like growth factors and their binding proteins in prostate cancer: cause or consequence? *Urologic Oncology*. 24 (4) 294-306.

Melnik BC, John SM, Carrera-Bastos P and Cordain L. 2012. The impact of cow's milk-mediated mTORC1-signaling in the initiation and progression of prostate cancer. *Nutrition and Metabolism*. 9 (1) 74.

Mellon M, Benbrook C and Benbrook KL. 2001. *Hogging It: Estimates of Antimicrobial Abuse in Livestock*. Washington DC: Union of Concerned Scientists.

Merritt RJ and Jenks BH. 2004. Safety of soy-based infant formulas containing isoflavones: the clinical evidence. *The Journal of Nutrition*. 134 (5) 1220S-1224S.

Messina M. 2010. Insights gained from 20 years of soy research. *The Journal of Nutrition*. 140 (12) 2289S-2295S.

Millar D, Ford J, Sanderson J, Withey S, Tizard M, Doran T and Hermon-Taylor J. 1996. IS900 PCR to detect Mycobacterium paratuberculosis in retail supplies of whole pasteurized cows' milk in England and Wales. *Applied and Environmental Microbiology*. 62 (9) 3446-3452.

Mills PK, Beeson WL, Philips RL and Fraser GE. 1989. Cohort study of diet, lifestyle, and prostate cancer in Adventist men. *Cancer*. 64 (3) 598-604.

Mills EJ, Rachlis B, Wu P, Devereaux PJ, Arora P and Perri D. 2008. Primary prevention of cardiovascular mortality and events with statin treatments: a network meta-analysis involving more than 65,000 patients. *Journal of the American College of Cardiologists*. 52 (22) 1769-1781.

Mishra S, Xu J, Agarwal U, Gonzales J, Levin S and Barnard ND. 2013. A multicenter randomized controlled trial of a plant-based nutrition program to reduce body weight and cardiovascular risk in the corporate setting: the GEICO study. *European Journal of Clinical Nutrition*. 67 (7) 718-724.

Moss, M. 2010. While Warning About Fat, U.S. Pushes Cheese Sales. New York Times, 6 November, 2010. Available from: www.nytimes.com/2010/11/07/us/07fat.html?pagewanted=all&_r=0 [Accessed 22 October 2013].

Monsanto, 2009. *rBST: a Safety Assessment* [online]. Available from: www.monsanto.com/newsviews/Documents/rbst_safety_assessment_071409.pdf [Accessed 18 September 2013].

Morimoto LM, Newcomb PA, White E, Bigler J and Potter JD. 2005. Variation in plasma insulin-like growth factor-1 and insulin-like growth factor binding protein-3: personal and lifestyle factors (United States). *Cancer Causes Control*. 16 (8) 917-927.

Morrison LM. 1960. Diet in coronary atherosclerosis. *The Journal of the American Medical Association*. 25, 173, 884-888.

Mortensen EL, Michaelsen KF, Sanders SA and Reinisch JM. 2003. Breast feeding and intelligence. *Ugeskrift Laeger*. 165 (13) 1361-1366.

Moss M and Freed D. 2003. The cow and the coronary: epidemiology, biochemistry and immunology. *International Journal of Cardiology*. 87 (2-3) 203-216.

Mowlem A. 2011. Goats. In: John Webster, 2011. *Management and Welfare of Farmed Animals. The UFAW Farm Handbook. Universities Federation for Animal Welfare*. Wiley Blackwell, p388.

Moynihan PJ, Wright WG and Walton AG. 1996. A comparison of the relative acidogenic potential of infant milk and soya infant formula: a plaque pH study. *International Journal of Paediatric Dentistry*. 6 (3) 177-181.

MRC/BHF, 2006. *MRC/BHF Heart Protection Study, questions and answers about cholesterol*. [online] Available at: www.ctsu.ox.ac.uk/~hps/fact_chol.shtml [Accessed 15 October 2013].

Munro IC, Harwood M, Hlywka JJ, Stephen AM, Doull J, Flamm WG and Adlercreutz H. 2003. Soy isoflavones: a safety review. *Nutrition Review*. 61 (1) 1-33.

Muntoni S, Cocco P, Aru G and Cucca F. 2000. Nutritional factors and worldwide incidence of childhood type 1 diabetes. *American Journal of Clinical Nutrition*. 71 (6) 1525-9.

Murphy N, Norat T, Ferrari P, Jenab M, Bueno-de-Mesquita B, Skeie G, Dahm CC, Overvad K, Olsen A, Tjønneland A, Clavel-Chapelon F, Boutron-Ruault MC, Racine A, Kaaks R, Teucher B, Boeing H, Bergmann MM, Trichopoulou A, Trichopoulos D, Lagiou P, Palli D, Pala V, Panico S, Tumino R, Vineis P, Siersema P, van Duijnhoven F, Peeters PH, Hjartaker A, Engeset D, González CA, Sánchez MJ, Dorronsoro M, Navarro C, Ardanaz E, Quirós JR, Sonestedt E, Ericson U, Nilsson L, Palmqvist R, Khaw KT, Wareham N, Key TJ, Crowe FL, Fedirko V, Wark PA, Chuang SC and Riboli E. 2012. Dietary fibre intake and risks of cancers of the colon and rectum in the European prospective investigation into cancer and nutrition (EPIC). *PLoS One*. 7 (6) :e39361.

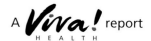

Murphy N, Norat T, Ferrari P, Jenab M, Bueno-de-Mesquita B, Skeie G, Olsen A, Tjønneland A, Dahm CC, Overvad K, Boutron-Ruault MC, Clavel-Chapelon F, Nailler L, Kaaks R, Teucher B, Boeing H, Bergmann MM, Trichopoulou A, Lagiou P, Trichopoulos D, Palli D, Pala V, Tumino R, Vineis P, Panico S, Peeters PH, Dik VK, Weiderpass E, Lund E, Garcia JR, Zamora-Ros R, Pérez MJ, Dorronsoro M, Navarro C, Ardanaz E, Manjer J, Almquist M, Johansson I, Palmqvist R, Khaw KT, Wareham N, Key TJ, Crowe FL, Fedirko V, Gunter MJ and Riboli E. 2013. Consumption of Dairy Products and Colorectal Cancer in the European Prospective Investigation into Cancer and Nutrition (EPIC). *PLoS One*. 8 (9) :e72715.

NACC, 2010. *Crohn's Disease* [online]. Available from: www.crohnsandcolitis.org.uk/Resources/CrohnsAndColitisUK/Doc uments/Publications/Booklets/Crohns Disease.pdf [Accessed 15 October 2013].

The National Board of Health (Denmark), 1998. *Recommendations for the nutrition of infants; recommendations for health personnel* [in Danish]. Copenhagen, Denmark: The National Board of Health (Denmark).

National Eczema Society, 2013. *What is eczema?* [online]. Available from: www.eczema.org/what-is-eczema [Accessed 17 September 2013].

National Eczema Society, 2013a. *Atopic eczema* [online]. Available from: www.eczema.org/atopic-eczema [Accessed 17 September 2013].

National Osteoporosis Society, 2013. *Key Facts & Figures* [online] Available from:www.nos.org.uk/page.aspx?pid=328 [Accessed 24 October 2005].

Newby PK, Tucker KL and Wolk A. 2005. Risk of overweight and obesity among semivegetarian, lactovegetarian, and vegan women. *American Journal of Clinical Nutrition*. 81 (6) 1267-1274.

Netherwood T, Martin-Orue SM, O'Donnell AG, Gockling S, Graham J, Mathers JC and Gilbert HJ. 2004. Assessing the survival of transgenic plant DNA in the human gastrointestinal tract. *Nature Biotechnology*. 22 (2) 204-209.

Newburg DS. 2000. Oligosaccharides in human milk and bacterial colonization. *Journal of Pediatric Gastroenterology and Nutrition*. 30 Suppl 2: S8-17.

NHS Choices, 2011. *Hay fever* [online] Available at: www.nhs.uk/conditions/hay-fever/pages/introduction.aspx [Accessed 17 September 2013].

NHS Choices, 2012. *Eight tips for healthy eating* [online] Available at: www.nhs.uk/Livewell/Goodfood/Pages/eight-tips-healthy-eating.aspx [Accessed 2 September 2013].

NHS Choices, 2012a. *Acne.* [online] Available from: www.nhs.uk/Conditions/Acne/Pages/Introduction.aspx [Accessed 13 September 2013].

NHS Choices, 2012b. *Atopic eczema* [online] Available from: www.nhs.uk/conditions/Eczema-%28atopic%29/ Pages/Introduction.aspx [Accessed 17 September 2013].

NHS Choices, 2012c. *Eczema: 7 tips to stop the itch.* [online] Available from: www.nhs.uk/Livewell/Allergies/Pages/Stopthescratching.aspx [Accessed 17 September 2013].

NHS Choices, 2012d. *Arthritis.* [online] Available from: www.nhs.uk/conditions/arthritis/Pages/Introduction.aspx [Accessed 17 September 2013].

NHS Choices, 2012e. *Lung cancer myths and facts* [online] Available from: www.nhs.uk/Conditions/Cancer-of-the-colon-rectum-or-bowel/Pages/Causes.aspx [Accessed 23 September 2013].

NHS Choices, 2012f. *Ovarian cancer* [online] Available from: www.nhs.uk/Conditions/Cancer-of-the-ovary/Pages/Introduction.aspx [Accessed 7 October 2013].

NHS Choices, 2012g. *Prostate cancer* [online] Available from: www.nhs.uk/Conditions/Cancer-of-the-prostate/Pages/Introduction.aspx [Accessed 9 October 2013].

NHS Choices, 2012h. *Causes of prostate cancer* [online] Available from: www.nhs.uk/Conditions/Cancer-of-the-prostate/Pages/Causes.aspx [Accessed 9 October 2013].

NHS Choices, 2012i. *Colic* [online] Available from: www.nhs.uk/conditions/colic/Pages/Introduction.aspx [Accessed 10 October 2013].

NHS Choices, 2012j. *Constipation* [online] Available from: www.nhs.uk/Conditions/Constipation/Pages/Introduction.aspx [Accessed 12 October 2013].

NHS Choices, 2012k. *Cardiovascular Disease* [online] Available from: www.nhs.uk/Conditions/cardiovascular-disease/Pages/Introduction.aspx [Accessed 14 October 2013].

NHS Choices, 2012l. *Can fish oil prevent heart attack deaths?* [online] Available from: www.nhs.uk/news/2012/10October/Pages/Fish-oil-could-save-thousands-of-women-from-heart-attacks-deaths.aspx [Accessed 14 October 2013].

NHS Choices, 2012m. *Diabetes, Type 2, causes* [online] Available from: www.nhs.uk/Conditions/Diabetes-type2/Pages/Causes.aspx [Accessed 17 October 2013].

NHS Choices, 2012n. *Middle ear infection (otitis media) - Symptoms* [online] Available from: www.nhs.uk/Conditions/Otitis-media/Pages/Symptoms.aspx [Accessed 19 October 2013].

NHS Choices, 2012o. *Gallstones* [online] Available from: www.nhs.uk/Conditions/gallstones/Pages/introduction.aspx [Accessed 19 October 2013].

NHS Choices, 2012p. *Gallstones – prevention* [online] Available from: www.nhs.uk/Conditions/Gallstones/Pages/Prevention.aspx [Accessed 19 October 2013].

NHS Choices, 2012q. *Migraine* [online] Available from: www.nhs.uk/conditions/migraine/pages/introduction.aspx [Accessed October 21 2013].

NHS Choices, 2012r. *Multiple sclerosis* [online] Available from: www.nhs.uk/conditions/multiple-sclerosis/pages/introduction.aspx [Accessed 21 October 2013].

NHS Choices, 2012s. *Obesity* [online] Available from: www.nhs.uk/conditions/obesity/pages/introduction.aspx [Accessed 22 October 2013].

NHS Choices, 2012t. *Osteoporosis* [online] Available from: www.nhs.uk/Conditions/osteoporosis/Pages/Introduction.aspx [Accessed 24 October 2013].

NHS Choices, 2012u. *Cancer* [online] Available from: www.nhs.uk/conditions/Cancer/Pages/Introduction.aspx [Accessed 7 January 2014].

NHS, 2012v. *Vitamins and minerals – Calcium* [online]. Available from: http://www.nhs.uk/Conditions/vitamins-minerals/Pages/Calcium.aspx [Accessed May 8 2014].

NHS Choices, 2013. *Food Labels* [online] Available from: www.nhs.uk/livewell/goodfood/pages/food-labelling.aspx [Accessed 17 September 2013].

NHS Choices, 2013a. *Lung cancer myths and facts* [online] Available from: www.nhs.uk/Livewell/Lungcancer/ Pages/Lungcancermythsandfacts.aspx [Accessed 23 September 2013].

NHS Choices, 2013b. *Eat less saturated fat* [online] Available from: www.nhs.uk/livewell/goodfood/pages/eat-less-saturated-fat.aspx [Accessed 14 October 2013].

NHS Choices, 2013c. *Lower your cholesterol* [online] Available from: www.nhs.uk/Livewell/Healthyhearts/Pages/Cholesterol.aspx [Accessed 14 October 2013].

NHS Choices, 2013d. *Crohn's Disease* [online] Available from: www.nhs.uk/Conditions/Crohns-disease/Pages/Introduction.aspx [Accessed 15 October 2013].

NHS Choices, 2013e. *Food poisoning* [online] Available from: www.nhs.uk/conditions/Food-poisoning/Pages/Introduction.aspx [Accessed 20 October 2013].

NHS Choices, 2013f. *Food poisoning -Causes* [online] Available from: www.nhs.uk/Conditions/Food-poisoning/Pages/Causes.aspx [Accessed 20 October 2013].

NHS Choices, 2013g. *Can I give my baby soya-based infant formula?* [online] Available from: www.nhs.uk/chq/Pages/can-I-give-my-baby-soya-based-infant-formula.aspx?CategoryID=62&SubCategoryID=63 [Accessed 10 February 2014].

NHS Direct Wales, 2013. *Crohn's Disease* [online] Available from: www.nhsdirect.wales.nhs.uk/encyclopaedia/c/article/crohnsdisease / [Accessed 15 October 2013].

NICE, 2011. *Otitis media with effusion* [online] Available from: http://cks.nice.org.uk/otitis-media-with-effusion#!topicsummary [Accessed 20 October 2013].

NICE, 2012. *NICE publishes new guideline on Crohn's disease* [online] Available from: www.nice.org.uk/newsroom/pressreleases/CrohnsDiseaseGuideline.jsp [Accessed 15 October 2013].

Nomura AM, Hankin JH, Henderson BE, Wilkens LR, Murphy SP, Pike MC, Le Marchand L, Stram DO, Monroe KR and Kolonel LN. 2007. Dietary fiber and colorectal cancer risk: the multiethnic cohort study. *Cancer Causes Control*. 18 (7) 753-764.

Norat T, Bingham S, Ferrari P, Slimani N, Jenab M, Mazuir M, Overvad K, Olsen A, Tjonneland A, Clavel F, Boutron-Ruault MC, Kesse E, Boeing H, Bergmann MM, Nieters A, Linseisen J, Trichopoulou A, Trichopoulos D, Tountas Y, Berrino F, Palli D, Panico S, Tumino R, Vineis P, Bueno-de-Mesquita HB, Peeters PH, Engeset D, Lund E, Skeie G, Ardanaz E, Gonzalez C, Navarro C, Quiros JR, Sanchez MJ, Berglund G, Mattisson I. Hallmans G. Palmqvist R. Day NE Khaw KT, Key TJ, San Joaquin M, Hemon B, Saracci R, Kaaks R and Riboli E. 2005. Meat, fish, and colorectal cancer risk: the European Prospective Investigation into cancer and nutrition. *Journal of the National Cancer Institute*. 97 (12) 906-916.

Nsouli TM, Nsouli SM, Linde RE, O'Mara F, Scanlon RT and Bellanti JA. 1994. Role of food allergy in serous otitis media. *Annals of Allergy*. 73 (3) 215-219.

Office for National Statistics, 2009. *Colorectal Cancer England 2009* [online]. Available from: www.ons.gov.uk/ons/rel/cancer-unit/bowel-cancer-in-england/2009/sum-colorectal.html [Accessed 25 September 2013].

Office for National Statistics, 2010. *Breast Cancer: Incidence, Mortality and Survival, 2010* [online]. Available from: www.ons.gov.uk/ons/rel/cancer-unit/breast-cancer-in-england/2010/sum-1.html [Accessed 25 September 2013].

Office for National Statistics, 2013. *Avoidable deaths from cardiovascular disease fell sharply between 2001 and 2011 in England and Wales* [online]. www.ons.gov.uk/ons/rel/subnational-health4/avoidable-mortality-in-england-and-wales/2011/sty-avoidable-mortality.html Available from: [Accessed 14 October 2013].

Ogle KA and Bullock JD. 1980. Children with allergic rhinitis and/or bronchial asthma treated with elimination diet: a five-year follow-up. *Annals of Allergy*. 44 (5) 273.

Ornish D, Brown SE, Scherwitz LW, Billings JH, Armstrong WT, Ports TA, McLanahan SM, Kirkeeide RL, Brand RJ and Gould KL. 1990. Can lifestyle changes reverse coronary heart disease? The Lifestyle Heart Trial. *The Lancet*. 336 (8708) 129-133.

Ornish D, Weidner G, Fair WR, Marlin R, Pettengill EB, Raisin CJ, Dunn-Emke S, Crutchfield L, Jacobs FN, Barnard RJ, Aronson WJ, McCormac P, McKnight DJ, Fein JD, Dnistrian AM, Weinstein J, Ngo TH, Mendell NR and Carroll PR. 2005. Intensive lifestyle changes may affect the progression of prostate cancer. *Journal of Urology*. 174 (3) 1065-1069.

Oski FA. 1985. Is bovine milk a health hazard? *Pediatrics*. 75 (1 Pt 2) 182-186.

Oski FA. 1996. *Don't Drink Your Milk*. New York: TEACH Services Inc.

Ostrowska L, Czapska D, Stefanska E, Karczewski J and Wyszynska U. 2005. Risk factors for cholecystolithiasis in obesity and at normal weight. *Roczniki Panstwowego Zakladu Higieny*. 56 (1) 67-76.

Outwater JL, Nicholson A and Barnard N. 1997. Dairy products and breast cancer: the IGF-I, estrogen, and bGH hypothesis. *Medical Hypotheses*. 1997 48 (6) 453-461.

Oxford University Hospitals NHS Trust, 2011. *BRCA1 and BRCA2 for men. Information for men from families with a known alteration in the BRCA1/2 gene* [online]. Available from: www.ouh.nhs.uk/patient-guide/leaflets/files%5C120417brca1brca2.pdf [Accessed 10 October 2013].

Owen CG, Martin RM, Whincup PH, Davey-Smith G, Gillman MW and Cook DG. 2005. The effect of breastfeeding on mean body mass index throughout life: a quantitative review of published and unpublished observational evidence. *American Journal of Clinical Nutrition*. 82: 1298-1307.

Pan A, Chen M, Chowdhury R, Wu JH, Sun Q, Campos H, Mozaffarian D and Hu FB. 2012. α-Linolenic acid and risk of cardiovascular disease: a systematic review and meta-analysis. *American Journal of Clinical Nutrition*. 96 (6) 1262-1273.

Park Y, Leitzmann MF, Subar AF, Hollenbeck A, Schatzkin A. 2009. Dairy food, calcium, and risk of cancer in the NIH-AARP Diet and Health Study. *Archives of Internal Medicine*. 2009. 169 (4) 391-401.

Parkin DM, Boyd L and Walker LC. 2010. Chapter 16. The fraction of cancer attributable to lifestyle and environmental factors in the UK in 2010. *British Journal of Cancer*. 105 Suppl 2: S77-81.

Paronen J, Knip M, Savilahti E, Virtanen SM, Ilonen J, Akerblom HK and Vaarala O. 2000. Effect of cow's milk exposure and maternal type 1 diabetes on cellular and humoral immunization to dietary insulin in infants at genetic risk for type 1 diabetes. Finnish Trial to Reduce IDDM in the Genetically at Risk Study Group. *Diabetes*. 49 (10) 1657-65.

Patelarou E, Girvalaki C, Brokalaki H, Patelarou A, Androulaki Z and Vardavas C. 2012. Current evidence on the associations of breastfeeding, infant formula, and cow's milk introduction with type 1 diabetes mellitus: a systematic review. *Nutrition Reviews*. 70 (9) 509-519.

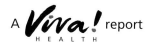

PCRM, 2005. *Doctors Group Files Suit against Kraft, General Mills, Dannon, and Dairy Trade Groups for False Dairy Weight-Loss Claims* [online] Available from: http://pcrm.org/media/news/doctors-group-files-suit-against-kraft-general [Accessed 22 October 2013].

Peters U, Sinha R, Chatterjee N, Subar AF, Ziegler RG, Kulldorff M, Bresalier R, Weissfeld JL, Flood A, Schatzkin A and Hayes RB; Prostate, Lung, Colorectal, and Ovarian Cancer Screening Trial Project Team. 2003. Dietary fibre and colorectal adenoma in a colorectal cancer early detection programme. *The Lancet.* 361(9368):1491-1495.

Petit HV. 2002. Digestion, milk production, milk composition, and blood composition of dairy cows fed whole flax seed. *Journal of Dairy Science.* 85 (6) 1482-1490.

Pickup RW, Rhodes G, Arnott S, Sidi-Boumedine K, Bull TJ, Weightman A, Hurley M and Hermon-Taylor J. 2005. Mycobacterium avium subsp. paratuberculosis in the catchment area and water of the River Taff in South Wales, United Kingdom, and its potential relationship to clustering of Crohn's disease cases in the city of Cardiff. *Applied and Environmental Microbiology.* 71 (4) 2130-2139.

Pietinen P, Malila N, Virtanen M, Hartman TJ, Tangrea JA, Albanes D and Virtamo J. 1999. Diet and risk of colorectal cancer in a cohort of Finnish men. *Cancer Causes and Control.* 10 (5) 387-396.

Pixley F, Wilson D, McPherson K and Mann J. 1985. Effect of vegetarianism on development of gall stones in women. *British Medical Journal.* 291 (6487) 11-12.

Pizzorno J, Frassetto LA, and Katzinger J. 2010. Diet-induced acidosis: is it real and clinically relevant? *British Journal of Nutrition.* 103 (8) 1185-1194.

Plant J. 2007. *Your life in your hands, understanding, preventing and overcoming breast cancer.* London: Virgin Publishing Limited.

Playford RJ, Woodman AC, Clark P, Watanapa P, Vesey D, Deprez PH, Williamson RC and Calam J. 1993. Effect of luminal growth factor preservation on intestinal growth. *Lancet.* 341 (8849) 843-848.

Playford RJ Macdonald CE and Johnson WS. 2000. Colostrum and milk-derived peptide growth factors for the treatment of gastrointestinal disorders. *American Journal of Clinical Nutrition.* 72, 5-14.

Post RE, Mainous AG 3rd, King DE and Simpson KN. 2012. Dietary fiber for the treatment of type 2 diabetes mellitus: a meta-analysis. *Journal of the American Board of Family Medicine* 25 (1) 16-23.

Pot GK, Prynne CJ, Roberts C, Olson A, Nicholson SK, Whitton C, Teucher B, Bates B, Henderson H, Pigott S, Swan G and Stephen AM. 2012. National Diet and Nutrition Survey: fat and fatty acid intake from the first year of the rolling programme and comparison with previous surveys. *British Journal of Nutrition.* 107 (3) 405-415.

Potter SM. 1995. Overview of proposed mechanisms for the hypocholesterolemic effect of soy. *The Journal of Nutrition.* 125 (3 Suppl) 606S-611S.

Pratt WB and Holloway JM. 2001. Incidence of hip fracture in Alaska Inuit people: 1979-89 and 1996-99. *Alaska Medicine.* 43 (1) 2-5.

Price AJ, Allen NE, Appleby PN, Crowe FL, Travis RC, Tipper SJ, Overvad K, Grønbæk H, Tjønneland A, Johnsen NF, Rinaldi S, Kaaks R, Lukanova A, Boeing H, Aleksandrova K, Trichopoulou A, Trichopoulos D, Andarakis G, Palli D, Krogh V, Tumino R, Sacerdote C, Bueno-de-Mesquita HB, Argüelles MV, Sánchez MJ, Chirlaque MD, Barricarte A, Larrañaga N, González CA, Stattin P, Johansson M, Khaw KT, Wareham N, Gunter M, Riboli E and Key T. 2012. Insulin-like growth factor-I concentration and risk of prostate cancer: results from the European Prospective Investigation into Cancer and Nutrition. *Cancer Epidemiology Biomarkers Previews.* 21 (9) 1531-1541.

Pringle H. 1998. Neolithic Agriculture: Reading the Signs of Ancient Animal Domestication. *Science.* 282, 1448.

Prosser CG, Fleet IR and Corps AN. 1989. Increased secretion of insulin-like growth factor I into milk of cows treated with recombinantly derived bovine growth hormone. *The Journal of Dairy Research.* 56 (1) 17-26.

Psaltopoulou T, Ilias I and Alevizaki M. 2010. The role of diet and lifestyle in primary, secondary, and tertiary diabetes prevention: a review of meta-analyses. *Review of Diabetic Studies.* 7 (1) 26-35.

Qin LQ, Wanf PY, Kaneko T, Hoshi K and Sato A. 2004. Estrogen: one of the risk factors in milk for prostate cancer. *Medical Hypotheses.* 62 (1) 133-142.

Ramsaransing GS, Mellema SA and De Keyser J. 2009. Dietary patterns in clinical subtypes of multiple sclerosis: an exploratory study. *Nutrition Journal.* 8, 36.

Rasinperä H, Savilahti E, Enattah NS, Kuokkanen M, Tötterman N, Lindahl H, Järvelä I and Kolho KL. 2004. A genetic test which can be used to diagnose adult-type hypolactasia in children. *Gut.* 53 (11) 1571-1576.

Rautiainen S, Levitan EB, Orsini N, Åkesson A, Morgenstern R, Mittleman MA and Wolk A. 2012. Total antioxidant capacity from diet and risk of myocardial infarction: a prospective cohort of women. *American Journal of Medicine.* 125 (10) 974-980.

Robinson S and Fall C. 2012. Infant nutrition and later health: a review of current evidence. *Nutrients.* 4 (8) 859-874.

Roddam AW, Allen NE, Appleby P, Key TJ, Ferrucci L, Carter HB, Metter EJ, Chen C, Weiss NS, Fitzpatrick A, Hsing AW, Lacey JV Jr, Helzlsouer K, Rinaldi S, Riboli E, Kaaks R, Janssen JA, Wildhagen MF, Schröder FH, Platz EA, Pollak M, Giovannucci E, Schaefer C, Quesenberry CP Jr, Vogelman JH, Severi G, English DR, Giles GG, Stattin P, Hallmans G, Johansson M, Chan JM, Gann P, Oliver SE, Holly JM, Donovan J, Meyer F, Bairati I and Galan P. 2008. Insulin-like growth factors, their binding proteins, and prostate cancer risk: analysis of individual patient data from 12 prospective studies. *Annals of Internal Medicine.* 149 (7) 461-471.

Royal College of Paediatrics and Health, 2013. *Breastfeeding figures fall as NHS budget is cut.* [online] Available from www.rcpch.ac.uk/news/breastfeeding-figures-fall-nhs-budget-cut [Accessed 12 September 2013].

Renehan AG, Painter JE, Atkin WS, Potten CS, Shalet SM and O'Dwyer ST. 2001, High-risk colorectal adenomas and serum insulin-like growth factors. *The British Journal of Surgery.* 88, 107-113.

Riordan AM, Hunter JO, Cowan RE, Crampton JR, Davidson AR, Dickinson RJ, Dronfield MW, Fellows IW, Hishon S and Kerrigan GN. 1993. Treatment of active Crohn's disease by exclusion diet: East Anglian multicentre controlled trial. *The Lancet.* 342 (8880) 1131-1134.

Rizos EC, Ntzani EE, Bika E, Kostapanos MS and Elisaf MS. 2012. Association between omega-3 fatty acid supplementation and risk of major cardiovascular disease events: a systematic review and meta-analysis. *Journal of the American Medical Association*. 308 (10) 1024-1033.

Robbins, J. 2001. *The Food Revolution, how your diet can help save your life and the world*. Berkeley, California, USA. Conari Press.

Rosell MS, Appleby PN, Spencer EA and Key TJ. 2004. Soy intake and blood cholesterol concentrations: a cross-sectional study of 1033 pre- and postmenopausal women in the Oxford arm of the European Prospective Investigation into Cancer and Nutrition. *American Journal of Clinical Nutrition*. 80 (5) 1391-1396.

Royal College of Physicians, 2003. *Containing the Allergy Epidemic*. London: Royal College of Physicians.

Ruhrah, J. 1909. The soy bean in infant feeding: preliminary report. *Archives of Pediatrics*. 26, 496-501.

Saarinen KM, Pelkonen AS, Makela MJ and Savilahti E. 2005. Clinical course and prognosis of cow's milk allergy are dependent on milk-specific IgE status. *Journal of Allergy and Clinical Immunology*. 116 (4) 869-875.

Sacks FM, Ornish D, Rosner B, McLanahan S, Castelli WP and Kass EH. 1985. Plasma lipoprotein levels in vegetarians. The effect of ingestion of fats from dairy products. *Journal of the American Medical Association*. 254 (10) 1337-1341.

Salque M, Bogucki PI, Pyzel J, Sobkowiak-Tabaka I, Grygiel R, Szmyt M and Evershed RP. 2013. Earliest evidence for cheese making in the sixth millennium BC in northern Europe. *Nature*. 493 (7433) 522-525.

Sartor RB. 2005 Does Mycobacterium avium subspecies paratuberculosis cause Crohn's disease? *Gut*. 54 (7) 896-898.

Savino F, Cresi F, Maccario S, Cavallo F, Dalmasso P, Fanaro S, Oggero R, Vigi V and Silvestro L. 2003. "Minor" feeding problems during the first months of life: effect of a partially hydrolysed milk formula containing fructo- and galacto-oligosaccharides. *Acta Paediatrica Suppl*. 91 (441) 86-90.

Savino F, Cresi F, Pautasso S, Palumeri E, Tullio V, Roana J, Silvestro L and Oggero R. 2004. Intestinal microflora in breastfed colicky and non-colicky infants. *Acta Paediatrica*. 93 (6) 825-829.

Savino F, Palumeri E, Castagno E, Cresi F, Dalmasso P, Cavallo F, Oggero R. 2006. Reduction of crying episodes owing to infantile colic: A randomized controlled study on the efficacy of a new infant formula. *European Journal of Clinical Nutrition*. 60 (11) 1304-1310.

Schwarz S and Leweling H. 2005. Multiple sclerosis and nutrition. *Multiple Sclerosis*. 11 (1) 24-32.

Scialla JJ and Anderson CA. 2013. Dietary acid load: a novel nutritional target in chronic kidney disease? *Advances in Chronic Kidney Disease*. 20 (2) 141-149.

Sechi LA, Scanu AM, Molicotti P, Cannas S, Mura M, Dettori G, Fadda G and Zanetti S. 2005. Detection and Isolation of Mycobacterium avium subspecies paratuberculosis from intestinal mucosal biopsies of patients with and without Crohn's disease in Sardinia. *The American Journal of Gastroenterology*. 100 (7) 1529-1536.

Segasothy M and Phillips PA. 1999. Vegetarian diet: panacea for modern lifestyle diseases? QJM: *Monthly Journal of the Association of Physicians*. 92 (9) 531-544.

Sellmeyer DE, Stone KL, Sebastian A and Cummings SR. 2001. A high ratio of dietary animal to vegetable protein increases the rate of bone loss and the risk of fracture in postmenopausal women. *American Journal of Clinical Nutrition*. 73 (1) 118-122.

Seppo L, Korpela R, Lonnerdal B, Metsaniitty L, Juntunen-Backman K, Klemola T, Paganus, A and Vanto T. 2005. A follow-up study of nutrient intake, nutritional status, and growth in infants with cow milk allergy fed either a soy formula or an extensively hydrolyzed whey formula. *American Journal of Clinical Nutrition*. 82 (1) 140-145.

Seppo L, Tuure T, Korpela R, Järvelä I, Rasinperä H and Sahi T. 2008. Can primary hypolactasia manifest itself after the age of 20 years? A two-decade follow-up study. *Scandinavian Journal of Gastroenterology*. 43 (9) 1082-1087.

Setchell KD and Lydeking-Olsen E. 2003. Dietary phytoestrogens and their effect on bone: evidence from in vitro and in vivo, human observational, and dietary intervention studies. *American Journal of Clinical Nutrition*. 78 (3 Suppl) 593S-609S.

Shingfield KJ, Bonnet M and Scollan ND. 2013. Recent developments in altering the fatty acid composition of ruminant-derived foods. *Animal*. 7 Suppl 1:132-62.

Shu XO, Zheng Y, Cai H, Gu K, Chen Z, Zheng W and Lu W. 2009. Soy food intake and breast cancer survival. *Journal of the American Medical Association*. 302 (22) 2437-2443.

Simonart T. 2012. Acne and whey protein supplementation among bodybuilders. *Dermatology*. 225 (3) 256-258.

Silveira MB, Carraro R, Monereo S and Tébar J. 2007. Conjugated linoleic acid (CLA) and obesity. *Public Health and Nutrition*. 10 (10A) 1181-1186.

Silverberg NB. 2012. Whey protein precipitating moderate to severe acne flares in 5 teenaged athletes. *Cutis*. 90 (2) 70-72.

Sinha R, Cross AJ, Graubard BI, Leitzmann MF and Schatzkin A. 2009. Meat intake and mortality: a prospective study of over a half a million people. *Archives of Internal Medicine*. 169 (6) 562-571.

Sirtori CR, Agradi E, Conti F, Mantero O and Gatti E. 1977. Soybean-protein diet in the treatment of type-II hyperlipoproteinaemia. *Lancet*. 1 (8006) 275-277.

Sirtori CR, Pazzucconi F, Colombo L, Battistin P, Bondioli A and Descheemaeker K. 1999. Double-blind study of the addition of high-protein soya milk v. cows' milk to the diet of patients with severe hypercholesterolaemia and resistance to or intolerance of statins. *British Journal of Nutrition*. 82 (2) 91-96.

Skoner AR, Skoner KR and Skoner DP. 2009 Allergic rhinitis, histamine, and otitis media. *Allergy and Asthma Proceedings*. 30 (5) 470-481.

SMA Careline. (sma.information@uk.nestle.com) February 11 2014. Re: *Reply from SMA Careline*. E-mail to J. Butler (justine@viva.org.uk).

Snowdon DA. 1988. Animal product consumption and mortality because of all causes combined, coronary heart disease, stroke, diabetes, and cancer in Seventh-day Adventists. *American Journal of Clinical Nutrition*. 48 (3) 739-748.

Soh P, Ferguson EL, McKenzie JE, Homs MY and Gibson RS. 2004. Iron deficiency and risk factors for lower iron stores in 6-24-month-old New Zealanders. *European Journal of Clinical Nutrition*. 58 (1) 71-79.

Song SH. 2012. Emerging type 2 diabetes in young adults. *Advances in Experimental Medical Biology*. 771: 51-61.

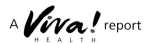
Speedy AW. 2003. Global production and consumption of animal source foods. *The Journal of Nutrition*. 133 (11 Supplement 2) 4048S-4053S.

Spock B and Parker SJ. 1998. *Baby and Child Care, the one essential parenting book*. London: Simon and Schuster UK Limited.

Stattin P, Rinaldi S, Biessy C, Stenman UH, Hallmans G and Kaaks R. 2004. High levels of circulating insulin-like growth factor-I increase prostate cancer risk: a prospective study in a population-based non-screened cohort. *Journal of Clinical Oncology*. 22 (15) 3104-3112.

Story L, Anderson JW, Chen WJ, Karounos D and Jefferson B. 1985. Adherence to high-carbohydrate, high-fiber diets: long-term studies of non-obese diabetic men. *Journal of the American Dietetic Association*. 85 (9) 1105-1110.

Strom BL, Schinnar R, Ziegler EE, Barnhart KT, Sammel MD, Macones, GA, Stallings VA, Drulis JM, Nelson SE and Hanson SA 2001. Exposure to soy-based formula in infancy and endocrinological and reproductive outcomes in young adulthood. *Journal of the Medical Association*. 286 (7) 807-814.

Swagerty DL Jr, Walling AD and Klein RM. 2002. Lactose intolerance. *American Family Physician*. 65 (9) 1845-1850.

Swank RL and Dugan BB. 1990. Effect of low saturated fat diet in early and late cases of multiple sclerosis. *Lancet*. 336 (8706) 37-39.

Swinburn BA, Caterson I, Seidell JC and James WP. 2004. Diet, nutrition and the prevention of excess weight gain and obesity. *Public Health Nutrition*. 7 (1A) 123-146.

Talbot G. 2006. *Independent advice on possible reductions for saturated fat in products that contribute to consumer intakes. Summary Report Prepared for Food Standards Agency* [online]. Available from: www.food.gov.uk/multimedia/pdfs/reductions.pdf

Tappel A. 2007. Heme of consumed red meat can act as a catalyst of oxidative damage and could initiate colon, breast and prostate cancers, heart disease and other diseases. *Medical Hypotheses*. 68 (3) 562-564.

Taylor EN, Stampfer MJ and Curhan GC. 2004. Dietary factors and the risk of incident kidney stones in men: new insights after 14 years of follow-up. *Journal of the American Society of Nephrology*. 15 (12) 3225-3232.

Taylor EN, Fung TT, Curhan GC. 2009. DASH-style diet associates with reduced risk for kidney stones. *Journal of the American Society of Nephrology*. 20 (10) 2253-2259.

TEDDY Study Group. 2008. The Environmental Determinants of Diabetes in the Young (TEDDY) Study. *Annals of the New York Academy of Sciences*. 1150, 1-13.

Terry P, Giovannucci E, Michels KB, Bergkvist L, Hansen H, Holmberg L and Wolk A. 2001. Fruit, vegetables, dietary fiber, and risk of colorectal cancer. *Journal of the National Cancer Institute*. 93 (7) 525-533.

Thomas HV, Key TJ, Allen DS, Moore JW, Dowsett M, Fentiman IS and Wang DY. 1997. A prospective study of endogenous serum hormone concentrations and breast cancer risk in post-menopausal women on the island of Guernsey. *British Journal of Cancer*. 76 (3) 401-405.

Thompson WG, Rostad Holdman, N, Janzow DJ, Slezak JM, Morris KL and Zemel MB. 2005. Effect of energy-reduced diets high in dairy products and fiber on weight loss in obese adults. *Obesity Research*. 13 (8) 1344-1353.

Thorsdottir I and Ramel A. 2003. Dietary intake of 10- to 16-year-old children and adolescents in central and northern Europe and association with the incidence of type 1 diabetes. *Annals of Nutrition and Metabolism*. 47 (6) 267-275.

Toohey ML, Harris MA, DeWitt W, Foster G, Schmidt WD and Melby CL. 1998. Cardiovascular disease risk factors are lower in African-American vegans compared to lacto-ovo-vegetarians. *Journal of the American College of Nutrition*. 17 (5) 425-434.

Trapp CB and Barnard ND. 2010. Usefulness of vegetarian and vegan diets for treating type 2 diabetes. *Current Diabetes Reports*. 10 (2) 152-158.

Tricon S, Burdge GC, Williams CM, Calder PC and Yaqoob P. 2005. The effects of conjugated linoleic acid on human health-related outcomes. *Proceedings of the Nutrition Society*. 64 (2) 171-182.

Trock BJ, Hilakivi-Clarke L and Clarke R. 2006. Meta-analysis of soy intake and breast cancer risk. *Journal of the National Cancer Institute*. 98 (7) 459-471.

Trowell H. 1974. Diabetes mellitus death-rates in England and Wales 1920-70 and food supplies. *The Lancet*. 2 (7887) 998-1002.

Tseng M, Breslow RA, Graubard BI and Ziegler RG. 2005. Dairy, calcium, and vitamin D intakes and prostate cancer risk in the national health and nutrition examination epidemiological follow-up study cohort. *American Journal of Clinical Nutrition*. 81 (5) 1147-1154.

Tucker KL, Olson B, Bakun P, Dallal GE, Selhub J and Rosenberg IH. 2004. Breakfast cereal fortified with folic acid, vitamin B-6, and vitamin B-12 increases vitamin concentrations and reduces homocysteine concentrations: a randomized trial. *American Journal of Clinical Nutrition*. 79 (5) 805-811.

Turck D. 2007. Soy protein for infant feeding: what do we know? *Current Opinion in Clinical Nutrional Metabolic Care*. 10 (3) 360-365.

Turner-McGrievy GM, Barnard ND and Scialli AR. 2007. A two-year randomized weight loss trial comparing a vegan diet to a more moderate low-fat diet. *Obesity (Silver Spring)*. 15 (9) 2276-2281.

Turunen S, Karttunen TJ and Kokkonen J. 2004. Lymphoid nodular hyperplasia and cow's milk hypersensitivity in children with chronic constipation. *The Journal of Pediatrics*. 145 (5) 606-611.

UK Parliament, 1999. *Select Committee on European Scrutiny Third and Fourth report, Use of Bovine Somatotropin (BST)*. [online] Available from: www.publications.parliament.uk/pa/cm199900/cmselect/cmeuleg/23-iii/2319.htm#n42 [Accessed 24 October 2013].

UNICEF, 2005. *Breastfeeding*. [online] Available from www.unicef.org/nutrition/index_24824.html [Accessed 12 September 2013].

UNICEF, 2013. *The UNICEF UK Baby Friendly Initiative – The health Benefits of breastfeeding*. [online] Available from www.unicef.org.uk/BabyFriendly/About-Baby-Friendly/Breastfeeding-in-the-UK/Health-benefits/ [Accessed 9 September 2013].

UNICEF, 2013a. *Breastfeeding – Impact on child survival and global situation*. [online] Available from www.unicef.org/nutrition/index_24824.html [Accessed 9 September 2013].

Vaarala O, Knip M, Paronen J, Hamalainen AM, Muona P, Vaatainen M, Ilonen J, Simell O and Akerblom HK. 1999. Cow's milk formula feeding induces primary immunization to insulin in infants at genetic risk for type 1 diabetes. *Diabetes*. 48 (7) 1389-1394.

Vehik K, Hamman RF, Lezotte D, Norris JM, Klingensmith GJ, Rewers M and Dabelea D. 2008. Trends in high-risk HLA susceptibility genes among Colorado youth with type 1 diabetes. *Diabetes Care*. 31 (7) 1392-1396.

Wahle KW, Heys, SD and Rotondo D. 2004. Conjugated linoleic acids: are they beneficial or detrimental to health? *Progress in Lipid Research*. 43 (6) 553-587.

Wakai K, Date C, Fukui M, Tamakoshi K, Watanabe Y, Hayakawa N, Kojima M, Kawado M, Suzuki K, Hashimoto S, Tokudome S, Ozasa K, Suzuki S, Toyoshima H, Ito Y and Tamakoshi A; JACC Study Group. 2007. Dietary fiber and risk of colorectal cancer in the Japan collaborative cohort study. *Cancer Epidemiology and Biomarkers Prevention*. 16 (4) 668-675.

Waldmann A, Koschizke JW, Leitzmann C and Hahn A. 2005. Dietary intakes and blood concentrations of antioxidant vitamins in German vegans. *International Journal for Vitamin and Nutrition Research*. 75 (1) 28-36.

Walsh, S. 2003. *Plant Based Nutrition and Health*. St. Leonard's-on-Sea, East Sussex. The Vegan Society.

Warensjö E, Byberg L, Melhus H, Gedeborg R, Mallmin H, Wolk A and Michaëlsson K. 2011. Dietary calcium intake and risk of fracture and osteoporosis: prospective longitudinal cohort study. *British Medical Journal*. 342: d1473.

WCRF/AICR, 2007. *Food, nutrition, physical activity, and the prevention of cancer: a global perspective* [online]. Available from: www.dietandcancerreport.org/cancer_resource_center/downloads/summary/english.pdf [Accessed: 27 September 2013].

WCRF, 2009. *Less than a third aware of processed meat cancer link*. [online] Available from: www.wcrf-uk.org/about_us/media/press_release.php?recid=64 [Accessed 7 January 2014].

Webster J. 2005. *Animal welfare; limping towards Eden*. Oxford: Blackwell Publishing Limited.

Weikert C, Walter D, Hoffmann K, Kroke A, Bergmann MM and Boeing H. 2005. The relation between dietary protein, calcium and bone health in women: results from the EPIC-Potsdam cohort. *Annals of Nutrition and Metabolism*. 49 (5) 312-318.

Whigham LD, Watras AC and Schoeller DA. 2007. Efficacy of conjugated linoleic acid for reducing fat mass: a meta-analysis in humans. *American Journal of Clinical Nutrition*. 85 (5) 1203-1211.

Whitmer RA, Gunderson EP, Barrett-Connor E, Quesenberry CP Jr and Yaffe K. 2005. Obesity in middle age and future risk of dementia: a 27 year longitudinal population based study. *British Medical Journal*. 330 (7504) 1360.

WHO, 2003. *Global strategy on diet, physical activity and health*. [online] Available from: www.who.int/dietphysicalactivity/media/en/gsfs_general.pdf [Accessed 5 September 2013].

WHO, 2003a. *Recommendations for preventing osteoporosis* [online] Available from: www.who.int/nutrition/topics/5_population_nutrient/en/index25.html [Accessed 24 October 2013].

WHO, 2006. *Chronic Disease, key risk factors include, high blood pressure, low fruit and vegetable intake*. [online] Available from: www.who.int/dietphysicalactivity/media/en/gsfs_chronic_disease.pdf [Accessed 14 October 2013].

WHO/FAO, 2002. *Diet, nutrition and the prevention of chronic diseases: Infancy 4.4.4*. [online] Available from: www.who.int/nutrition/topics/4_dietnutrition_prevention/en/index1.html [Accessed 14 October 2013].

WHO, 2005b. *Obesity and overweight*. [online] Available from: www.who.int/dietphysicalactivity/publications/facts/obesity/en/ [Accessed 31 October 2005].

WHO, 2013. *Infant and young child feeding - Fact sheet N°342*. [online] Available at: www.who.int/mediacentre/factsheets/fs342/en/index.html [Accessed 9 September 2013].

WHO, 2013a. *Breast cancer: prevention and control* [online] Available at: www.who.int/cancer/detection/breastcancer/en/index1.html [Accessed 25 September 2013].

WHO, 2013b. *Diabetes Fact sheet N°312* [online] Available from: www.who.int/mediacentre/factsheets/fs312/en/index.html [Accessed October 17 2013].

WHO, 2013c. *General information related to microbiological risks in food*. [online] Available from: www.who.int/foodsafety/micro/general/en/print.html [Accessed 20 October 2013].

WHO, 2013d. *Mean Body Mass Index (BMI)* [online] Available from: www.who.int/gho/ncd/risk_factors/bmi_text/en/ [Accessed 22 October 2013].

WHO, 2013e. *Overweight and obesity. Fact sheet N°311* [online] Available from: www.who.int/mediacentre/factsheets/fs311/en/index.html [Accessed 22 October 2013].

Wickham CA, Walsh K, Cooper C, Barker DJ, Margetts BM, Morris J and Bruce SA. 1989. Dietary calcium, physical activity, and risk of hip fracture: a prospective study. *British Medical Journal*. 299 (6704) 889-892.

Wieneke AA, Roberts D and Gilbert RJ. 1993. Staphylococcal food poisoning in the United Kingdom, 1969-90. *Epidemiology and Infection*. 110, 519-531.

Willer CJ, Dyment DA, Risch NJ, Sadovnick AD and Ebers GC; Canadian Collaborative Study Group. 2003. Twin concordance and sibling recurrence rates in multiple sclerosis. *Proceedings of the National Academy of Sciences*. 100 (22) 12877-12882.

Willetts IE, Dalzell M, Puntis JW and Stringer MD. 1999. Cow's milk enteropathy: surgical pitfalls. *Journal of Pediatric Surgery*. 34 (10) 1486-1488.

Williams G and Pickup J. 2004. *Handbook of Diabetes*. Massachusetts, US: Blackwell Publishing.

Wilmot EG, Davies MJ, Yates T, Benhalima K, Lawrence IG and Khunti K. 2010. Type 2 diabetes in younger adults: the emerging UK epidemic. *Postgraduate Medical Journal*. 86 (1022): 711-718.

Winzenberg T, Shaw K, Fryer J and Jones G. 2006. Effects of calcium supplementation on bone density in healthy children: meta-analysis of randomised controlled trials. *British Medical Journal*. 333 (7572) 775.

Wolk A, Mantzoros CS, Andersson SO, Bergstrom R, Signorello LB, Lagiou P, Adami HO and Trichopoulos D. 1998. Insulin-like growth factor 1 and prostate cancer risk: a population-based case-control study. *Journal Of The National Cancer Institute*. 90, 911-915.

Wolk A. 2005. Diet, lifestyle and risk of prostate cancer. *Acta Oncologica*. 44 (3) 277-281.

Wosje KS and Kalkwarf HJ. 2004. Lactation, weaning, and calcium supplementation: effects on body composition in postpartum women. *American Journal of Clinical Nutrition*. 80 (2) 423-429.

Wu AH, Pike MC and Stram DO. 1999. Meta-analysis: dietary fat intake, serum estrogen levels, and the risk of breast cancer. *Journal of the National Cancer Institute*. 91 (6) 529-534.